TAKE ME

OR

HEAL ME

An Ultimatum
From a Weary Heart

a memoir

RINAD BSHARAT

AVIVA
PUBLISHING
NEW YORK

TAKE ME OR HEAL ME:
An Ultimatum From a Weary Heart

ISBN 978-1-63618-107-3 (paperback)

ISBN 978-1-63618-145-5 (hardcover)

Library of Congress Control Number 2021916421

Any Internet addresses and phone numbers printed in this book are offered as a resource. They are not intended in anyway to be or imply an indorsement by Aviva, nor does Aviva vouch for the content of these sites and numbers for the life of this book.

Printed in the United States

1st edition • November 2021

Aviva Publishing
2301 Saranac Avenue
Lake Placid, NY 12946
518-523-1320

www.avivapubs.com

Dedication

This book is dedicated to three of the most amazing women in my life: my mom, Nihad, my Aunt Ellen, and my sister, Loren. I would not have survived this long without your love, support, and guidance. You all have given me strength, urging me to fight each day. Thank you for believing in me, praying for me, loving me, and mostly for teaching me to love all my imperfections. Mama, you taught me about God and asked each day to "meet me at His feet." Because of that, I have learned to live in His love and know I am never alone. You nurtured me from kitten to tiger and taught me what strength really means. Aunt Ellen, you are the strongest and most resilient person I know, taking each day with a smile and looking at the best in every situation. You taught me that adversity does not define us but rather it strengthens us and lifts us to a higher purpose. Loren, you are my best friend, and the voice reminding me to fight. You gave me the tough love I never wanted but always needed. To know you is to love you.

Mom and Dad, you taught your children the most important life lessons. You taught us to have integrity, to always live in faith and hope, and to believe God is in control. As kids, we learned these lessons by watching you both live this way every day. You instilled the confidence in each of your kids to aim for the stars. Baba, you showed me that any child of yours has nothing to fear.

To my amazing husband, Bertrand, you make me want to be the best version of myself and you love me "a million" even when I fall short. You are the partner I wanted and waited for, and I am forever grateful you are in my life. We are in this together.

Table of Contents

Author's Note

This story, at its heart, is an atypical love story.

When I started writing, I thought this book was about my search for a cure. I wanted to share how I navigated this scary and complicated journey and hoped others could benefit from my hindsight and diligent research. Writing was my salvation from the frightening world of chemo and radiation and all things cancer-related. It became my soapbox, my way to tell the world of all the challenges I encountered at such a young age.

Then it became about finding the love of my life, the partner and spouse I wanted to share this journey with for however long I got to walk the earth. Dating seemed such an all-encompassing part of my life when I was first diagnosed at twenty-three so it was only logical I would write about it. Surely someone else loving me would provide a calm haven within the storm, ease my fears, and help me bear the weight of this burden.

Somewhere along the way, I discovered that what I really wanted was to find my relationship with God. Only by recognizing that control of my future truly rested in the hands of God could I find peace in the unknown. Acknowledging His love and His strength would guide me through the difficult decisions and help me accept that I was not being punished. I had been chosen for this path by God in His infinite wisdom, and even if I never knew why, there was a reason behind it.

But the truth of the matter is, my story is about learning to love myself. For all the confidence I may exhibit to the world, there is an uncertain young girl inside wondering if she's doing the right thing—giving up on medical school, refusing a marriage proposal, moving to a new city, standing up against a doctor who made a mistake. All of these choices created doubts in my mind.

My story is about finding the love of my life (I did!) and discovering my strength through a strong relationship with God. But both of those only became possible when I started to love and trust myself. I could not give to my future spouse and to God what I did not give to myself—learning this lesson made so many things possible for me.

It would be great if learning that lesson meant the work was over, but it doesn't. Love is always changing—and it is challenged daily, so it must learn to adapt. The good news, however, is that God's love is forever.

In that strength and love, I am also forever.

INTRODUCTION

The Ultimate Catch-22

"You know the situation, Rinad," he said, looking as serious as I'd ever seen him. "I believe the only thing that can save you now is a bone marrow transplant. I think you should begin the testing for marrow immediately."

I shook my head.

"If you do not follow the regimen I've prescribed, I can't continue to be your doctor. It's my opinion that you won't live more than three months as things are now." I could tell it was hurting him to say this as much as it was for me to hear it.

Then he turned and walked out of the room.

✝

My name is Rinad Bsharat and I should be dead by now. In March 2005, I was told I had three months to live. Yet it is 2021, and I am still here.

For more than fifteen years, I have been on a toxic journey with Hodgkin's Lymphoma, and through this time, I have racked up three fatal diseases, each of which on their own kill people every day. I need three different transplants to survive: a bone marrow transplant to cure the cancer, and lung and heart transplants to address damage done during my cancer treatments. But my heart and lungs are too weak for the bone marrow transplant, and I won't be approved for an organ transplant while I still have cancer. To top it off, the antirejection medicines required after any of the transplants run the risk of giving me lymphoma.

My entire existence is a Catch-22.

CHAPTER 1

Woman Plans and God Laughs

As a girl, obviously I never imagined I would have cancer for eighteen years and counting. I imagined I would go to school, have a successful career, get married, maybe have children. I thought I would host dinner parties, go ice skating, and take my kids trick-or-treating, going through life one sunny moment after another. I thought those things . . . until I got my diagnosis in August 2003, when I was twenty-three years old. And then I didn't have those thoughts anymore. Those dreams were just too painful, so I had to let them go.

Don't get me wrong. I grew up and built an adult life, and some aspects are normal. I have a wonderful family I see as often as possible, filled with adorable nieces and nephews. I am active in my church. I have two careers that I enjoy juggling. But life hasn't always been like that and it has largely been punctuated by chemo and chronic fatigue, existential crises, and nights when I would fall asleep wanting nothing more than to wake up cured or dead.

Take me or heal me, I would pray.

Neither has happened yet.

Along the chaotic and lonely journey, though, I now see this was all part of God's plan for me. I'm just along for the ride.

Maybe this memoir is different from others. Maybe it's not. Most are written after the author has overcome their great obstacle, but I'm not yet cured. I'm in the midst of my ninth life now, waiting for the conclusion to this fight. I can say that, as I walk through this story, one blaring truth remains consistent: I have spent my life teetering back and forth over an invisible line—as an Arab girl living in America, a Christian girl with a weak understanding of what it means to be a child of God, and a sick girl who is on the brink of dying but who does not actually die. Will I finally find the real me?

CHAPTER 2

She'll Be Coming 'Round the Mountain When She Comes

Since I was a little girl, my father has called me *Bisseh*, the Arabic word for cat. It is tradition in Arabic cultures for a person to have multiple nicknames, or *teknonyms*, honorifics in place of, or alongside, given names. These names can refer to the bearer's first-born child or sometimes a familiar characteristic. They are given with respect and love by those closest to the person.

Similarly, my mom named her four children based on their varied personalities. My older brother, the eldest of us all, had to step in a lot as the man of the house since my father worked hard and couldn't spend much time at home. Because of this, my mom called him "Lion." Loren was the social one, the type of person whom you would be compelled to tell your life story to as soon as you met her. She was bold and brash at times, but always humorous and friendly. She liked to include everybody in the conversation but had a way of making you feel like the only person in the room when she talked to you. Loren was fittingly dubbed "Butterfly." Baby Danny was "Eagle," since he was the only one born in America and, with three very type-A older siblings, had to learn to soar above all the nonsense.

To my mother, I was "Tiger."

When I was younger, I would ask my mother why she called me that. "You will have to find out for yourself," she would always reply. "One day, that name will help you understand yourself better."

As usual, my mother was right. Tigers, though meek as cubs, grow to be strong and fearless. I was a submissive child, always following my parents' orders, even when I did not agree with them.

From a very young age I did not want to cause trouble or be branded a troublemaker. One time, my friends decided they wanted candy right before a church service. They knew the pastor kept some behind the lectern, so they snuck some a few minutes before services started. Even though our parents were chatting with other adults, not paying attention, I would not join in the act and refused to take some of the spoils. They were stolen goods and I did not want to be associated with them. I knew the second the candy touched my lips, my parents would somehow know, and I would forever be known as a thief and troublemaker.

It took some time for my stripes to fully show, to grow into my own.

There were a lot of ways *Bisseh* fit me as a child as well. I'm particular, lithe and intelligent, picky about the company I keep, and prone to strong moods and even stronger opinions. I am a perfectionist.

I like it that way.

It is what has made me successful. I am usually punctual and great at multitasking, taking advantage of every moment and maximizing my productivity. I have always hated wasting time except, as my mother likes to joke, when it came time to be born.

It was a cold December day in Mafraq, Jordan when my mom went into labor with me in 1979. She was by herself, her belly swollen to its limits, so late in her pregnancy that she had been put on bedrest. The doctors said she was due any day but that the baby was *taking her time*. That might be the only time in my life I ever procrastinated.

My dad was working, my oldest brother was at school, and my grandmother had taken my sister to the neighbor's house to play. My mom stayed behind, hoping to sneak in a short afternoon nap. As she rose from the bed, she felt the familiar pains of labor and realized it was time. Stuck at home alone, Mom made her way to the phone in the kitchen and called the midwife. I was born thirty minutes later. I may have procrastinated the arrival, but once I decided it was time, I didn't delay!

My mom delivered me in the middle of the cold kitchen floor. The midwife who assisted was older and very respected in Mafraq. She had delivered hundreds of babies. But when I was born, Mom said I was so rosy the midwife gave me a kiss before handing me to her. This was unusual, but she explained that I was so flush, so full of new life, that she had not been able to resist.

I fit the nickname *Bisseh* in another way, the way a name given sometimes foretells someone's life—a prophecy.

I would also have nine lives.

That's how many different cancer treatments I have pursued, with the expectation that each would be the last time. Each reoccurrence, I am told I am on the brink of being cured or dying—both bringing equal measures of hope and fear.

Every relapse has felt like an ending, each remission another reincarnation, another life for *Bisseh*. But for many years, I wasn't really alive. I was just going through the motions, waiting for something to free me from this strange purgatory. Will my fight be over this time? Has the cat lived her last life? I have lived those years like the watch on my wrist, with every minute and hour that passes by ticking precariously, wondering when the gears would jam, when that faint tick would cease, and silence would fall upon me at last.

Life in this world is full of unknowns, variables we cannot see, events and circumstances for which there are no formulas to deduce their meaning. Throughout this battle, the tormenting cycle has been the same. I get sick, get treatment, get better, and then get sick again. Every time the cancer metastasizes, I ask myself the same questions: What am I supposed to learn from this? Who am I supposed to become? What does God have in store for me?

I have tried many things to cope with these unending and never-answered questions over the course of my journey. I've gone from relying solely on faith, to questioning God completely. I've tried Zen meditation and I've tried nothingness. I've undergone every medical intervention, traditional and natural, practicing every state of mind, hoping something, anything, would stick. But nothing has. When I was left completely alone with just my illness—no faith or God to guide me to the end, whether that was life or death—that was the worst. That was when I was at my lowest.

When I think about my dance with this disease, I can't help but think of Moses and Mt. Sinai. When the Israelites were freed from bondage in Egypt, Moses was sent by God to lead them to the Promised Land. Along their way through the wilderness, they began to doubt God. The Israelites whined and complained as they roamed through the desert. They did everything *but* trust God, though miracles happened before their very eyes, conveying God's promise to them. And because of this doubt, the journey took forty years rather than eleven days. Their punishment for their lack of faith was circling the same mountain for four decades!

Here I am in my second decade, circling the same mountain of *Cancer*, looking for my Promised Land. I keep enduring and waiting, and just when I think I've finally shaken it, the cancer comes back into my life.

And every time, doubt creeps into my mind.

For the longest time I thought, like the Israelites, I was being punished by God for my lack of faith. Was my disobedience responsible for the constant recurrence of my cancer? Or if not that, was I supposed to learn a lesson and only then find healing?

I spent the better part of two decades searching for love, for a cure, and for God in all this darkness. The answer may not have been what I wanted or expected, but it was there nonetheless.

I just wasn't listening.

I created a new identity in the often-chaotic world of medicine and gave myself the labels I wanted rather than the labels put upon me. I didn't start this journey with three deadly diseases, but this is the path I'm walking now. It's always a new fight. The medicines are new. The trials are new. The doctors, the opinions, the hopes and fears—they change with every new obstacle and you never know if something will work. Survival is often about adaptation—just ask Charles Darwin—but sometimes all it does is buy you time until the next new thing comes along.

CHAPTER 3

Daddy Killed the Easter Bunny

Everyone likely struggles with their identity to some degree. But it's important to understand where my identity crisis started, which was crucial in developing my personality during my formative years, so you can fully appreciate my story.

For me, the confusion started early. I emigrated with my family from Jordan when I was still a baby. My parents brought with them the cultural norms for Jordanian families—especially those for Jordanian women. They had strict rules for what my sister and I were allowed to do. Not so many rules for my brothers, however.

This double standard often made me angry. If two people are faced with the same situation, the same rules should apply. As adults, we know that's not always the case, but it's sometimes hard to put that belief or desire aside, whether we're talking about curfews or the outcome of cancer treatment.

There were few people of color in the well-to-do neighborhood of Harrison, New York, where I attended school. English was my second language when I started kindergarten; we spoke Arabic at home. So that helped make me more of an outsider. Luckily, my mom was an English teacher, so I had a head start.

Nobody in our school looked like me and my family, so I was a bit confused about where I fit in. The American culture is a hodgepodge of ethnicities, languages, and belief systems, but fitting in is especially important in America. Some might call it conforming, but to a child who is already different from the other children around her, being seen as the same has its appeal.

Fitting in is also important when you're fighting for your life. There are very narrow criteria for clinical trials and new medications, and sometimes not fitting in can mean the difference between the chance at life, or death.

But back to kindergarten . . .

There was a group of Japanese-American girls in my class and I quickly joined them because we all had one thing in common: we were different from the other kids. Our golden-brown skin and foreign accents stood out against our classmates' light-colored hair and neutral speech.

We shared our differences with the same ease that other kids shared their peanut butter sandwiches with the crusts cut off. In my developing mind, I began to believe I was Japanese. Until my older sister, Loren, broke the news to me one afternoon as I tried on the new kimono I'd gotten for Christmas.

"You know you're not really Japanese, right?" She scoffed as only an older sister can.

I was shocked by the revelation, but quickly nodded. "Yeah, I know. I'm just pretending."

But inside I was screaming, *How can that be true*? I did all of the things my Japanese friends did. If I spoke Japanese and wore Japanese clothing and played with Japanese children, surely that meant I was Japanese. They accepted me. It took many months before the reality truly settled in.

As I grew older, the duality of my life compounded this identity crisis. At home, I lived in a protected circle my Jordanian parents created for their Jordanian daughters, while letting my brothers enjoy the freedoms of America. All around me, my friends went to sleepovers and hung out at the mall or the movie theater. I was only allowed out with my sister, and even that was extremely restricted by my parents' rules. What was expected of me did not match what was expected of my peers. While they were learning to figure out the world around them, I was preoccupied with finding my place in it.

It made me angry. Not so much about the rules themselves, but about the inconsistency and double standards. My brothers were able to pick and choose which cultural standards applied to them. I was not, and as I got older, my parents tightened the reins even further. The problem was, I was a perfectionist at my core. I was a diligent student. I was expected to obey, and obey I did.

I did not rebel against the strict curfews or even push the boundaries. Even without the curfews, I would have wanted to stay home and study. I didn't want to disturb the general peace of our family. Any strife would have made me anxious and distracted me from my studies. But I often wondered what it would have been like to live as my friends did. What secrets did my friends whisper in the dark between sleeping bags? What adventures did they have at the mall, meeting boys, trying on clothes or jewelry? Sometimes it made me sad, but I always reminded myself what really mattered: the freedom that awaited with college.

So even as a young child, I was looking ahead. Following the rules would get me a better prize down the road. Sure, it meant sacrificing sleepovers with friends and weekends hanging out, but once I was on my own in college, I could do what I wanted.

✝

It wasn't all bad growing up with Jordanian parents. Some parts were actually comical.

My father, whom we call Baba, was very enthusiastic in learning to fit into his new American home. He learned to see the opportunity and blessing in this new country, letting the homesickness and discomfort subside. My parents became American citizens as quickly as possible, adopting American holidays and the traditions that accompanied them.

Christian holidays in Jordan are not commercial affairs. They center around the birth and death of Jesus, celebrated exclusively by Christians. There was no Santa Claus or reindeer for Christmas, or bouncing bunnies in bow ties on Easter. In the United States, holidays have evolved into more secular and inclusive affairs, celebrated by people of all religions.

Although it was new to him, Baba loved the *Hallmark* aspect of the American culture. We exchanged candy and flowers on Valentine's Day, ate turkey for Thanksgiving, and watched fireworks on the 4th. My dad's birthday is March 16, and he looks forward to the corned beef and cabbage dinner my mom makes to celebrate every year.

Easter was particularly special because of our faith. My dad would always celebrate it with religious gusto, but this now included the American traditions. We didn't always understand every element of the way Americans celebrated the holidays, but this did not stop my father from lovingly preparing an Easter holiday surprise for the whole family. We had an Easter egg hunt, wore the pastel dresses we bought at JC Penney to church, and then concluded festivities with a lovely Easter supper.

I vividly remember one of our earlier Easters in America. My dad sat us around the table and reminded us of all our blessings, as we normally did before a meal. Then he proudly lifted up the cover to reveal the main dish—a plump bunny that was skinned, gutted, stuffed, roasted, and presented center table for dinner. When my father happily reported we were having rabbit, my siblings and I were shocked. We had been inundated with images of cute cartoon rabbits everywhere we went, and the idea of eating one was unthinkable.

Danny was hit the hardest. He burst into tears, shouting, "You killed the Easter Bunny!" over and over again.

Of course, who could blame my dad? When he heard there was an "Easter Bunny," he made the only logical assumption: In Jordan, there were no silly rabbits in bow ties, leaving candy-filled eggs for children to collect in faux grass-lined baskets. Rabbits, like lambs, were meant to be eaten, not dressed up and paraded around.

It may seem like a leap, but logical assumptions were a part of my thinking throughout my initial fight against cancer. Follow the rules. Listen to the doctors. Take the toxic medicines. Ignore what my body was telling me. Get the cure. Because the prize I was fighting for was not just freedom.

It was surviving.

✝

My first encounters with cancer were not my own. My mom's eldest sister married a Scottish man who had died from cancer several years before my own battle began. He was my favorite uncle growing up. I remember as a child he would let me sit on his lap and tug on his beard. His sparkling blue eyes twinkled as he laughed. He was a gentle and jovial man who passed too soon and suffered greatly. My parents were deeply affected by his untimely death, and concluded that cancer was simply something you died from and no other alternative was possible.

Subsequently, while in her junior year of college, my sister began showing unusual symptoms, including excessive itching that left her arms raw from scratch marks. Loren went to countless doctors, enduring test after test, but it was a long road to diagnosis. It wasn't until she saw a trained lymphoma specialist that we finally received the earth-shattering news: my sister had Hodgkin's Lymphoma, a type of blood cancer of the lymph nodes. If detected early, Hodgkin's is usually curable with a dozen rounds of chemotherapy and radiation.

Loren was in her final semester of college when she was diagnosed. Her classmates and friends rallied behind her and made sure she got her assignments and homework turned in on time. They helped her get extensions when she needed them. It was amazing to see such a strong support network around her; so many people cared about her during her illness. Her school administration was able to accommodate her special needs and she graduated on time.

Her diagnosis was a scary time for us because we'd already seen how this story ended for my uncle. Although they never stopped fighting for her, my parents internally prepared themselves for what they thought was inevitable. It was a very somber time in our household. My dad specifically had a hard time with the diagnosis, bursting into tears every time she entered the room. After the fourth or fifth time, my brothers and I would look at one another, each thinking, "Awkward!"

My sister would soon dismantle the belief in the *inevitable*. After seven months of treatment, Loren was cured and has been in remission since 2000. She is now married and has three happy, healthy boys. God was watching over her and our family.

I believed to my core when Loren was sick that God was with us. We prayed, we had faith in the doctors and the treatments. We were diligent with the rules. And at the end, Loren was granted a cure.

But the whole ordeal that galvanized the family also scarred us in the process. The death of my aunt's husband had taught us nobody survives cancer, and then Loren's cancer showed us that cancer was very curable. I think that explains why, when I was first diagnosed, my family didn't really take it that seriously. Loren followed the recommended treatment once diagnosed and she was easily cured. Well, maybe not easily, but cured nonetheless.

She followed the rules. She received her cure.

Her life, and that of the family, went back to normal.

Normal for me meant focusing on graduating college. I already saw college as the prize for my dedication to following the rules. In my mind, I'd sacrificed all the fun my friends had experienced in high school, so it was really important to maintain my grades to keep my scholarship so all the sacrifices wouldn't be in vain.

✝

I always knew if I wanted to attend college, it would have to be a great one. Harrison is an affluent suburb that dripped with elitism, and Ivy League schools were the norm. My parents did not shy away from that expectation. They were not going to send me to an institution with weak academics or a reputation for its party atmosphere, nor was that what I wanted for myself.

In the Arab culture, you are only as successful as your children. Parents are known to sacrifice for their kids, but their delayed gratification is rewarded with their childrens' life choices: who they marry, what profession they choose, if they have kids (read: boys), how financially successful they are.

Knowing this, I doubled down and spent every spare moment in high school studying for the SATs and my regular class exams so I could attend a boast-worthy university. On top of the assigned homework, I did supplemental reading for each of my classes, scheduled sessions with the teachers, and brought some of the outside information I learned into class discussions. In addition to regular school, my siblings and I attended Arabic school on Saturday mornings, where we learned how to read and write Arabic. As if we did not have enough assignments from our regular classes, they piled on more homework over the weekend.

The world was full of information. Why just limit myself to what one person wanted me to learn? To one perspective? Surely the more information you had the better, correct? Cats are curious, after all. If there was an avenue for me to improve my chances at a great college, I took it. I was again focused on the future, on the prize my dedication to following the rules would get me.

I'd known I wanted to go to college in the Washington, DC area for some time. My parents and I had become citizens when I was in second grade. Even at that young age, I knew what a tremendous opportunity I was granted and that it should not be taken lightly. In eighth grade, our class took a field trip to Washington, DC, and as soon as I stepped off the bus, I knew that was where I wanted to study. It was the center of our country's government, the place where laws were written and enforced, the place where big decisions were made. More importantly, the people who made the big decisions were there.

When I received the crisp, white envelope with The George Washington University stamped on the front, I could barely contain myself through my excitement and nerves. I ran inside, screaming for my mother, tore the envelope open, and paused, holding the folded letter in my hand. *The second I read this*, I thought, *my life will change, forever.*

I unfolded the letter with trembling hands. "Dear Miss Bsharat," I read aloud. "Congratulations! It is with great pleasure. . . . "

I couldn't even finish before my mother and I both began to cheer. We called for my father and siblings who came and rejoiced with us.

"Congratulations, Bisseh!" they said. "We knew you could do it!"

My hard work had paid off. More importantly, following the rules had paid off. It was one of the most surreal moments of my life. Here I was, a first-generation Arab-American, born on a kitchen floor in a small Jordanian village, and I had just been accepted into my first-choice university. I was getting my freedom!

College was a series of new lessons for me. I had convinced myself I wanted to become a doctor, even though I had a weak stomach. I just assumed that all med students blanched at the sight of blood in the beginning and that it was trained out of them as part of their education. Since I had a lot of Advanced Placement credits coming in as a freshman, I had the option of graduating college a year early. I'd started college early, at the young age of seventeen, so I would be eligible to graduate at twenty. I decided twenty was way too young to be out in the real world, so I elected to double major—Biology on a pre-med track, and Public Health and Health Services—to earn more credits and justify spending another year away.

My parents were proud of my choice of majors and allowed me to continue on the chosen track. I spent four years working as a medical assistant at various medical departments in The George Washington Hospital and The George Washington's School of Medicine. I had been accepted into a special work-study program where I could rotate between different departments with the medical students. It was a great opportunity, but my queasiness never subsided and I was not able to fully enjoy the opportunity.

I couldn't stand the graphics and photos in class, much less the sight of actual blood or organs during dissections. Many times, I felt like I would get sick or pass out, but I continued on, insistent that one day I would get over it. I found it somewhat strange that very few of the other students reacted the same way, but I brushed it off. I just had to follow the program and I would be like them in no time, I convinced myself. *Follow the rules, Bisseh.*

I vividly remember my first day in the surgical ward. I was tasked with helping a doctor with a case of necrotizing fasciitis, a flesh-eating disease. The doctor instructed me to hold the man's leg up so the nurse could scrub the dead flesh from his leg and bind it in a bandage. I have never come so close to vomiting on another human being.

Believe it or not, that wasn't the last straw. During my final year, I was doing a rotation in the OB/GYN ward. A woman in labor came in, and as I helped her onto the examination table, her water broke and spilled amniotic fluid all over my shiny white Keds. It was more than I could bear. I had stuck it out through necrotizing fasciitis, but this was somehow too much! I still find this amusing and a little disconcerting when I remember how I came to that decision.

It was a hard realization that medicine was not for me. I was such a perfectionist and had always been taught never to quit, no matter how hard the task. My dad expected a lot from his kids, whereas my mother was more intuitive and wanted us to thrive where we were comfortable. There would be many nights in the Bsharat household where you would hear my father's bellow throughout the cramped apartment. "Mistakes are for stupid people!" I will be the first to admit that, although it was unconventional, his militant form of discipline was effective. All four of us have advanced degrees and are successful in our own rights.

Quitting, like making mistakes, is for stupid, weak people, and I was neither. What would have happened if my parents had quit their efforts to build a life in America because it was hard? We would likely be back in Jordan, hiding from persecution, trying to survive each day.

✝

The Iranian Revolution, also known as the Islamic Revolution, had erupted in February 1979, and was raging on when I was born ten months later. Fear quickly swept across the Middle East that the revolution would spread into surrounding countries. If it reached Syria, Lebanon, or Jordan—collectively known as the Levant—it would mean persecution for my Christian family. As a religious minority in Jordan, we had never been afforded equal protection and opportunity under the law. Since our last name means *gospel* or *good news*, there was no hiding it. King Hussein and Queen Noor believed in being fair to Christians, but there was still much discrimination and there was no telling what would happen if the revolution crossed our borders.

In the middle of 1980, when my uncle was laid off from his job as an airline pilot without any reason, my parents knew it was just the beginning. The wave was slowly encroaching, and my family had to get out. My mother immediately started making plans to get her family onto a plane to New York.

Her escape plan also included her younger sister, Ellen, who had contracted polio as an infant and been left physically disabled. My aunt was ignored and marginalized in Jordan and my mother had the insight to know that she could live to her full potential in America. She wanted us to live in a place where people were given the same opportunities regardless of race, religion, gender, class, or disability.

When she learned that my father had to finish his tour in the Royal Jordanian Air Force and could not move with his family, she told him, "You can meet us in New York. That is where we will be," and handed him an address. My mother, her sister, and we three kids left a week later.

Right before we were supposed to leave Jordan, I got a bad case of tonsillitis. I was only six months old, and the doctors warned my mother that my health was fragile and I would not survive the journey to America. I only got worse in the days leading up to the flight, and the infection brought me close to death, despite the fact that I was taking the prescribed Erythromycin. My mother agonized over the decision but, ultimately, put her faith in God to see us through and get us on that plane to New York; and sure enough, He did.

We arrived in New York safely, and I was immediately taken to another doctor who discovered I was allergic to Erythromycin. The doctor in Jordan had not thought to test for the allergy. Instead of getting better, I got worse when they doubled my dosage. I was being poisoned. The American doctors changed the antibiotic, and I was fine within five days. That was my first brush with death, and the first time American doctors had saved me from it. But it would not be the last time I was poisoned by carelessness.

Our arrival in America was not glamorous. There was no big house, big car, or big TV. Life did not look the way it looked on *Happy Days*. We were in a country that was better off than our home country, and we had liberties and opportunities we could not have imagined as Christians in Jordan, but we certainly were not living the high life.

Regardless, my mother's decision was firm. She wanted to give her children a good life, and she was not going to let anything get in the way. If we had a little less than others, so be it; at least we had opportunity for more.

She had ignored everyone who second-guessed her decision to take us to America—the doctors who told her I might not survive the journey, and her parents who warned her how hard it would be, even temporarily, as a single mother in a foreign country. She'd made up her mind to succeed and she would not be swayed.

I am very much like my mother in that regard. Once I make a decision, I work hard and persevere until I succeed. This is why it was incredibly difficult for me to admit that something—med school, for example—was not a good fit for me. In my mind, I was simply not trying hard enough to make it work. The word *failure* played over and over again in my head and the perfectionist in me rebelled at the thought. I'd made a choice. I had to stick it out in medical school.

My second major required me to take master's-level courses in the School of Public Health, which opened my eyes to the massive shift happening in the health care system with the inception of Health Maintenance Organizations, or HMOs for short. Doctors no longer had the final say in how to practice medicine; the insurance companies are now negotiating patient care. This shift has caused major inefficiencies in the health care system. I decided I wanted to effectuate change from the inside. I just did not know what that looked like yet.

After much reflection, I decided it was time to alter my path. I wouldn't be a doctor, but my interest in making the medical system better for patients was a worthwhile pursuit. I was not failing—I was simply moving in a new direction, fine-tuning the journey toward my ultimate destination.

That I could live with.

CHAPTER 4

Arab Wife Training

After I graduated from college, I returned to my parents' house to begin sorting out my life. Meanwhile, my parents were focused on another area of my future.

While I was in college, even stretching back to my final years of high school, they were busying themselves doing what all good Arab parents do—finding my future husband. If you think building a new career path from the rubble of an old one is difficult, think about how much worse it is when you have suitors coming to the house inquiring about your life goals and five-year plan.

Over the previous four years, I had met no more than twelve prospective matches. These introductions happened often because my parents had two single daughters living at home. On a dozen occasions, random uncles twice removed called my parents trying to broker a meeting for marriage with their sons. My parents, gracious hosts that they were, would never turn away a guest, so every time a prospective suitor called, my parents willingly opened their home to these families.

Like most young girls who grew up watching Disney cartoons, I thought I would meet my soulmate and get caught up in a breathtaking, whirlwind romance. I expected to see this man and my heart would beat and butterflies would flutter in my stomach, and I would just know he was The One. It would be love at first sight, and we would be a perfect match for each other. I would love everything about him. There would never be any compromising or fighting, or any little thing about him that would annoy me. It was divinely ordained that this person would be my other half. He would be perfect. We would live happily ever after.

At the very least, I hoped I would have a fairy tale, love-at-first-sight instant attraction like my grandparents.

My grandmother, or Taita as we called her, was originally from Syria. With pale skin, auburn hair, and piercing green eyes, she was a good-looking young woman by any standard. When she was about fourteen years old, she and her father went to her elder sister's house to celebrate her wedding. It was a small Christian community, so my grandfather and his family were also in attendance. He saw my grandmother from a distance and was immediately smitten by her. Like a true Arab of that time, he recognized it would be taboo to approach her directly, but he knew he had to marry her.

Having no other choice, my grandfather "Googled" my grandmother the old-fashioned way, by simply asking about her around the village. Having found sufficient information, mainly her family name and address, he went over to her parents' house and declared to her father his intention to marry her. My great-grandfather was almost heartbroken at having to turn him away, as my grandmother's marriage to one of her cousins had already been planned.

Taita, however, was no complacent woman. The man to whom she was betrothed was a simple farmer. Meanwhile, this new suitor standing before her was not only very handsome, but also a prominent businessman. Wanting more out of life, she married him in the nearby village to avoid a spectacle with her cousin's family, and to keep the civility and respect between the families.

When her cousin found out that my grandmother eloped, he was furious. Of course, he couldn't just let them go without an old-fashioned show of his masculine prowess; he confronted my great-grandfather. How dare he allow an outsider to steal away his bride! He demanded an answer. My great-grandfather explained that his daughter was not kidnapped or coerced into marriage, but went of her own volition and was married in a church by a priest with witnesses.

Still unbelieving, the cousin tracked down the priest and demanded to hear the details from the clergyman himself. Finally, he was satisfied. My grandparents moved and established themselves ten miles away in Mafraq, what is present-day Jordan. They chose this location because of its thriving economy, and my grandfather, ever the intelligent businessman, needed to move where his business would strive. They bought a house and immediately started a family. They were living the Jordanian dream.

I'm not saying I want the same type of dalliance my grandparents had, but I would at least like to be the one to choose whom I spend my life with. I had a list, and I did not want a love story that started with, "and then he came over with his dad."

My dream husband would always be thoughtful and kind. This man would be well Americanized but, like me, have immigrant parents. He'd be able to relate to the cultural issues I faced growing up. He *could* be an Arab, but it was far more important that he be a Christian. He would bring flowers for his mother-in-law when we visited my parents, as he would never dream of arriving anywhere as a guest empty-handed. His parents would have taught him very well.

He would also be ambitious, financially stable, and able to take care of his family. He would lend and not borrow, and most of all, be gracious and generous to others. He would be humble in his actions, and would have integrity, something I valued highly because of the lessons instilled by my Baba.

My dad recently told me a story about a time he worked at the local gas station on the weekends. It was his second job because working one was not enough to feed a family of seven. He would often receive tips for pumping gas, but at the end of every shift, he would include his tips along with the cash he collected for the gas and hand it to the owner.

At the end of every shift, his manager noticed my dad would give more money back than was owed. His boss usually had the opposite problem. Other employees would short the owner, but with my dad, he made more money. On several occasions, the owner explained that the tips were for my father to keep, but my father insisted it was not his business and therefore not his money, and he refused to keep it. The owner trusted my dad and hired him to supervise the others. My dad, with his broken English, had earned the title of boss. They say girls always end up with someone like their father, and I hoped it would be true for me after hearing that story.

I know what you are thinking. "Rinad, your list of requirements for a husband is ridiculous! You'll never find someone like this!" I know. But hey, I'm not the first person to be disillusioned about love. I had never dated before (strict parents, remember?) and only had TV, movies, and romantic books on which to base my expectations. I didn't get any remotely realistic ideas until my college friends gave them to me, and even those were unreasonable for me.

I had gained much freedom with my departure to college except in this one area: I was not allowed to date and meet men organically. I was expected to have my *Mr. Right* introduced to me in a staged meeting at my parents' discretion. My notions of romance were as manufactured as a Valentine's Day teddy bear holding a heart-shaped box of chocolates from CVS.

If I'd enrolled in medical school, I would have had an acceptable excuse for not marrying so young and could reject any offers for suitors to come over. Now that I'd decided against medical school, I could not rely on this excuse.

Still, since all my siblings had married people with foreign parents—South American, Southeast Asian, and European—I thought I would simply fall in line. And I *wanted* to. I wanted someone who could relate to having immigrant parents. I wanted to meet the expectations of my parents in at least that small way.

My parents were worried, and justifiably so. I had just returned home from college with no plan and little direction. Months prior, I had decided I couldn't be a doctor—I was too squeamish. I had never given up on anything. My parents and I also knew I couldn't be a traditional Arab wife because I was becoming too bold and argumentative. I felt like a failure and I was heartbroken. I was angry and frustrated with myself. I felt like I had wasted my time, and I was at a complete loss for how or in what direction to move forward.

Little did I know, God had a longer-term plan for me.

After seeing the line of suitors my father had arranged for visits, I knew this wasn't the right path for me.

It so happened that while I was in college, a guy saw me at a wedding I attended with my parents during summer break. The following week he showed up at our house with his parents, uncle, and brother, as well as the bride from the wedding we had all attended. My parents, ever the welcoming couple to their daughter's suitors, received them into our living room and they all sat down. My father looked expectantly at the father of the suitor to state the purpose of their visit, although it was obvious to everyone present.

I could not have been more uninterested with the whole situation. I knew I was not going to marry the guy; I was just a freshman in college and was in no way ready to get married. I wanted to finish my studies.

The guy's father went on to say, "We saw you at the wedding and have found that you are a good family of credible standing in the community, and we want your youngest daughter for our son."

Yes, that is what he said. It might have lost a few words in the translation, but that was the gist of it. *He wanted me for his son.* Luckily, my father agreed with me. He told the suitor's father I was already enrolled in college and could not get married until I finished.

I thought that was the end of this particular family. However, about three years later, the guy's younger brother also saw me and my sister at yet another wedding. This time around, I did not have the excuse of college because I'd graduated two months earlier, and my parents were ready for me to settle down like a good Jordanian daughter. When the younger brother and his father arrived, my mother insisted that both of us dress in our prettiest clothes and host the guests properly.

Even though I was still not ready to get married, I did as my parents expected; my sister and I served the guests like we had been instructed. The suitor's father said to my father, "Both of your girls seem like they are educated and smart and also firmly rooted in the Middle Eastern culture. We'll take either one."

When I heard what he had said, I was outraged at his audacity. I was so incensed that I finally found my tongue in front of my parents, but of course waited until the guests left before voicing my opinion. I told them in no uncertain terms that if in the future anyone came inquiring at our house about me, they should either say I was already married or "tell them I'm dead."

Little did I know how much my bad joke would foreshadow the future.

However, the cat had finally grown into the tiger, and the tiger had grown into her stripes. I was the youngest daughter in an Arabic household and my place was to follow the guidance of my parents on all things, especially when it came to choosing a husband. These traditions had been handed down to and followed by—quite successfully, I'll admit—the women in our family for generations.

But I wanted my parents to know I was done being just a Jordanian girl. I'd tried the Jordanian way and followed the advice of my family on choosing my future husband. Those customs and traditions, however well they'd worked for my parents and might work for other members of my family, didn't work for me. I put my foot down. I was an American now.

I didn't do this lightly or without thought. I knew my actions could possibly hurt my parents' feelings, and that was the last thing I wanted. I respected and trusted them. But I knew what was best for me. This was at the very core of who I was as a person.

My parents agreed, much to my surprise. They were outraged at the way that guy's father had talked about their daughters. That was the last time an introduction was made for either of us.

After this incident, I knew I needed to get out and make my own way. But I had a problem. Even though I was legally an adult by American standards, I wasn't allowed to move out of my parents' home unless I either got married or went back to school—another pair of Jordanian cultural handcuffs. I had already tried the latter and lived in Washington, DC for four years, but because I nixed the plan on moving forward in medicine, my post-grad options were quite limited. I saw no apparent opportunity to move out any time soon. I needed to make one.

It's easy at this point if you are reading this to say, "But you are an adult. There is no legal way your parents could hold you to their customs about marriage or moving out on your own." And you would be mostly correct. But the ties of cultural expectations are deeper than legalities. I was raised with the belief that honoring my parents' wishes was the ultimate respect. They were my highest authority and I could no more go against them than I could decide to ignore gravity.

✝

The hardest part was figuring out a new career that my parents would not object to, and one I would actually enjoy. I browsed tons of graduate school brochures, scanning all the different programs and options. *The graduate school for business at NYU looks nice*, I considered, *or maybe the MBA program at the University of Michigan*. I frequented the library to read about the different courses and to see if any caught my interest. A few stood out, but none were enough to send me back into the mindset in which I lived my whole life—driven by a cosmic calling, a goal I could devote myself to fully. I spent all my time and energy on the search.

One night, I fell fast asleep atop a pile of graduate school brochures. I dreamed I was sitting in a lecture hall; it was familiar and comforting after spending most of the last four years in ones like it. I tried to hear the professor. His words were muffled and distant at first, but slowly they became clear, and I discovered I was in a law class. I woke up at 4 a.m., unable to think of anything else. That was it! Then and there I decided I would become a lawyer.

That morning, when I came downstairs to my family, I had a pronounced spring in my step. My heart felt light for the first time since returning home. I was going to go to law school. I finally had a plan and a future to work toward.

This is the part of the story where all the heroine's dreams come true, and everything is perfect again, and she lives happily ever after. My parents were happy, and because of that, I was more than happy. I had it all, almost. I still held on to the dream of meeting someone at law school who would sweep me off my feet. I was only twenty-two at this point and hadn't had a real boyfriend yet. I was living near New York City and had the world at my feet. During the day, I worked at a law office and prepared to take the LSAT. By night, I gallivanted around the city, enjoying everything it had to offer my friends and me. I was living the dream life of any girl in her early twenties.

Little did I know, I *would* be swept off my feet ... just not by a man.

CHAPTER 5

The Contiki Cough

It started with my inquisitive nature.

Ever the curious cat, with three grueling years of law school looming ahead, I wanted to get away from New York. I had always dreamed of exploring the glamorous cities of Europe, seeing all their beauty and culture. I craved adventure and wanted to get out and experience it before I was confined to a library where monotonous reviews of briefs and rulings would consume my life for the next three years.

I came across a website called Contiki, a company that hosted European tours. Beautiful, smiling, young adults from all over the world screamed at me from the computer screen. Lifelong friendships! Unlimited partying! Adventurous! Experience different cultures! It seemed like the perfect segue into the next chapter of my life. So, I signed up, and a short time later, I set out on an eight-week adventure that could more accurately be described as a glorified foreign frat party. Every detail of that brochure rang true. I made friends from Australia on that trip whom I still speak to on a regular basis.

We visited England, Spain, Italy, Greece, France, Germany, Belgium, Switzerland, and Austria, dancing the night away, every night. My typical day saw me getting up, bleary-eyed, my voice hoarse from all the talking, shouting, singing, and sitting in smoky bars. The European air in the early 2000s was essentially second-hand smoke. Then I would get on a bus to the next fabulous location and use the bus ride as an opportunity to sneak in a nap. I didn't want to miss a moment of action when we unloaded the bus. At night, we went out and socialized until almost dawn, then made our way back to the hotel and attempted to sleep for a few hours before doing it all over again. Europeans eat late and socialize even later, relying on a siesta to get through each day. We were determined to *do as the Romans do*.

The long days and nights did not, however, lend themselves to a particularly healthy lifestyle. Due to the nomadic nature of the trip, there was little access to nutritious, wholesome food, so my fellow travelers and I made do with fried snacks, entire loaves of bread filled with cheese, and copious amounts of wonderfully delicious European chocolate. Needless to say, our immune systems were primed for illness.

The Contiki staff had seen this all before and warned us about burning the candle at both ends, but we were young with endless energy and optimism and did not listen. Eventually, the partying lifestyle took its toll, but it ended up being much more than I bargained for.

With more than fifty people crammed into the tour bus—always together, breathing all over each other—when one person got sick, so did the rest. An outbreak of flu with a nasty cough spread through the entire party. We called it the "Contiki Cough."

I caught it, like everyone else, and like everyone else, I was miserable. But beyond it ruining a few days of the adventure, I wasn't really worried about it. After all, the symptoms were the same for everyone. The nagging cough, fatigue, night sweats, and fever—they seemed like normal signs of the virus. And when the night sweats did not go away, I chalked it up to being in Italy in the middle of summer with no air conditioning. But everyone else got better. I didn't.

I couldn't trick myself anymore. I was nervous, and all I could think about was Loren and all she had gone through a few years earlier. I broke down and consulted a fellow traveler who was a trained EMT; he put some of the worries out of my mind. He told me the worst thing I could have with these symptoms was mono. Still, there was this nagging feeling that would not go away. I tried my best to move on and salvage what I could from the rest of the trip, until I woke up from a two-hour nap and found an eight-centimeter mass protruding from my neck.

By the time I returned to the United States from my European grand tour in early June 2003, I was feeling worse than ever. Each day, my condition deteriorated. I was set to begin law school in two short months, but this new life of independence I had worked so hard to achieve seemed to be slipping away.

To make matters worse, I couldn't even see a doctor. I had to wait three months until I started law school to be added to my mother's insurance plan. If I had a serious diagnosis when enrolled on her plan, it would be classified as a preexisting condition, and the insurance company would not cover it.

Ah, the great American health care system.

Life #1

CHAPTER 6

Lightning Doesn't Strike Twice, or Does It?

I often wonder how different my life might have been had I not taken that trip to Europe. I had ignored a few good reasons to cancel the trip, like the impending war in 2003 in Iraq and the anti-American (and anti-Arab) sentiment that came with it. Most of Europe saw the United States' actions in the Middle East as self-serving. I actually looked into canceling the trip, but unfortunately, the contract was non-refundable. I had grown up in a household that was always careful with cash, so as I considered my options, I decided not to waste the money. Away I went.

The word *cancer* pinged around my brain. The memories of Loren's diagnosis and that of my uncle were never far from my thoughts. But what was the likelihood that two sisters would come down with cancer? Hodgkin's Lymphoma isn't thought to run in families, although siblings of young people with this disease have a higher risk. It's thought that a similar childhood exposure to certain infections or a shared inherited gene may play a part.

Besides, if I got checked right away, I would be sick *and* broke. Therefore, I suffered in silence. I did everything I could to hide the symptoms from my family due to the insurance situation. I didn't want them to worry and I knew they would insist on taking me to a doctor right away. My own fears played a big part in this as well. They say ignorance is bliss. It may not be bliss, but sometimes it beats the alternative.

But I could only take so much. I broke down and went to the doctor, deciding I would steer the conversation toward getting a prescription for antibiotics. *Unfortunately*, I had a doctor who could not be distracted by any other possibilities related to the mass protruding from my neck and smaller ones under my arm. I watched his face contort with confusion as he examined me.

As he scribbled the prescription for antibiotics, he told me point-blank, "If the mass and cough do not go away after taking these pills, you have cancer."

You are probably thinking this is the part of the story where the protagonist hears the word *cancer,* races home, falls on their knees, and prays to God that it be anything but *that.*

That's not what I did.

At this point, I still did not believe cancer was a real option. It couldn't be. I had followed all the rules, and God honors people who honor the rules. Although I didn't have a close relationship with God, there was no way He would let this happen to me.

But I felt a pang of fear stabbing my heart. Surely my sister honored the rules, as did my uncle. They were good people, but still got sick. What was happening here? Could I actually have the big C? I left the office appearing stoic, but wracked with fear and in obvious denial. Even so, I continued hiding my symptoms. Until one day when I didn't see my mother step into my room while I was on the phone. She let out a scream, then stood frozen, pointing at the golf ball sized lump protruding from my neck, unable to say a coherent word. My pretense was over.

Against my protests, my mother told my sister, who made me an appointment with her oncologist, Dr. S. When she told him the details of my condition, he told her, "Lightning doesn't strike twice." He didn't sound overly concerned that I might have cancer and thought it was most likely a bad case of mono. Infectious mononucleosis is caused by the Epstein-Barr Virus (EBV), but people who have had mono have a slightly increased risk of Hodgkin's Lymphoma, and he wanted me to come in and see him to confirm.

This left my mother and sister somewhat reassured. I wanted to feel that way, but there was something inside of me that was doubtful of the oncologist's assurance. I pushed the feeling down and tried my best to be light-hearted and positive, focusing on my future. I was going to law school. I was going to graduate and practice law. I would find love and be successful and happy. I would have a family and a career. I'd done everything the right way. *That* was my future, not cancer.

But when I went to see Dr. S the next day, his evaluation changed my rosy outlook. He examined the mass bulging from my neck and found similar ones under my arms. I tried to stay upbeat during the examination, cracking jokes to lighten the mood and break some of the tension. I'll never forget how this angered him.

He turned to me, his eyes narrow under his furrowed brow. "I don't think you understand how dangerous this could be," he chastised.

My stomach sank at his cross words. I did recognize the seriousness of my presence in his office, perhaps more than even he did. But I wasn't prepared mentally to accept a cancer diagnosis at that moment. Denial is not just a river in Egypt, as they say.

But I also didn't need my doctor berating me for coping in the way I thought best until I was prepared to deal with the news. In hindsight, ignoring the truth did not make my fight against the disease easier or faster. However, much as I did with my parents as authority figures, I didn't want to cause strife, so I bit my tongue.

At 7:30 the next morning, I got a call from Dr. S' office to come in for additional testing and was sent for an X-ray and PET scan. It was an agonizing two-day wait before being called back in to go over the results. On August 3, 2003, I was diagnosed with Stage 3B Hodgkin's Lymphoma. The cancer had started in my neck and had already spread down into my stomach. Dr. S wanted to confirm it had not spread to my bone marrow, which would make it Stage 4, and performed a bone marrow biopsy. This is a very painful procedure which consists of pushing a needle shaped like a corkscrew through my bone in my lower back under local anesthesia to aspirate a small amount of the marrow. The biopsy came back clear and I was diagnosed with Stage 3. The "B" referred to the fever and night sweats, which were aggressive cancer symptoms I exhibited.

My time in ignorance was over.

Oddly enough, the first feeling I had after hearing the diagnosis was annoyance. I'd rented an apartment in the city. I'd made my security deposit and paid my non-refundable fee for a three-year law school commitment. Didn't my body know I had plans?

Didn't God know I had plans?

It's important to understand my relationship with God at this point. It had never been too deep since I was, perhaps like most young Christians, immature in my faith. I believed in God, but I took His presence in my life for granted, somewhat like you take for granted the presence of your grandparents. You visit on the major holidays, share phone calls at the important moments, but on a day-to-day basis, they are not an active part of your life. But when you need them, they show up.

My parents had a more personal connection to God. They always relied on prayer to carry them through the tough times, and praised Him through the good ones. I'd seen them turn to God and to their faith when Loren was diagnosed. I remembered their words, "God will see us through," when times were tough.

They tried to raise their children in the Christian faith with all their Jordanian traditions and values, but while we attended church on Sunday, it never really stuck. Living in a country that was home to a variety of religions and cultures—even denominations within Christianity—I didn't understand the intricacies my faith had to offer.

Which is why, after leaving my parents' home for college, I stopped going to church. I saw attending church as a cultural mandate and only went on the major holidays when I was visiting home. That was pretty much the extent of my *being religious*.

I did not pray often before June 2003, with the exception of my sister's battle with the disease, because I never needed or wanted anything so badly that I needed to pray. I sailed through high school, went to the college of my first choice on scholarship, and graduated cum laude. My parents did a great job of sheltering us from the harsher realities of life.

Now, I tapped into the tenuous ties of faith between God and myself. I believed. I had no reason to doubt that my faith and good works would be rewarded. He would see me through to a cure. I believed the amount of suffering one endured was directly proportionate to how good of a person they were. Seeing I was no angel, but no devil either, a cure was quickly within my future.

Buoyed by this, and the knowledge that my sister beat this disease in seven months, I decided I'd do no less. This would be merely an inconvenience to my carefully planned life. I had played by the rules all my life and that had netted me a prestigious undergraduate degree. I would do the same here, and in less than a year, this would become nothing more than a memory, a story Loren and I would share at holidays in years to come. Dying did not cross my mind; I just wanted to get the treatments and move on with my life. Just with a new hairstyle.

No one in my family took my diagnosis too seriously. They were thinking the same thing —Loren's cancer was curable; therefore, mine was too. The biggest worry on all of our minds was the non-refundable deposit I had paid for law school, and how taking a year off would derail my plans.

The prescribed treatment was a cocktail of twelve cycles of ABVD—Adriamycin, Bleomycin, Vinblastine, and Dacarbazine. It's funny how they use the word cocktail, as if you are to believe you are lying on a beach somewhere having the time of your life. This was a textbook treatment, but not without its dangers. The Adriamycin portion is notorious for causing heart problems, specifically cardiomyopathy, which is a hardening of the heart muscle that can lead to heart failure. Bleomycin is linked with a lung condition called pulmonary fibrosis. Definitely not the pina colada I would want to order.

The side effects from this "B" in the mixture are so common that Lance Armstrong declined to take the very same treatment when he was diagnosed with cancer, fearing any damage to his lungs would end his cycling career. Before I began the treatment, I took a Pulmonary Function Test and had an echocardiogram to get baseline readings of my heart and lungs. Both came back within the normal limits. Aside from my bulging lymph nodes and hacking cough, I was perfectly healthy and a good candidate for the treatment.

That made me hopeful. In my mind I made a list: follow the treatment, feel badly in the short term, be free of cancer in the end. It seemed quite simple when you looked at it like that. I also saw the combination of cancer treatment and law school much like I perceived my preparations during high school to get into a top-tier college. I would do whatever extra work was necessary to see my plan to fruition and reach my goal.

But Dr. S was adamant I not attend law school during chemotherapy. He said a full-time law program would be too stressful on my weakened body. The first year of law school is notorious for weeding out students not cut out for the rigorous program.

Law school, for me, was more than getting a law degree. It was maintaining my independence.

And there was the money at stake. My family was comfortable, but that had not always been the case. My father often worked multiple jobs when I was a child to provide for our family, and we were taught the value of money.

The more I grew, the more I came to know we barely had enough money for our family of seven. I got my sister's hand-me-downs, which had come from our cousins, which had come from other more distant family members before them. I knew my parents couldn't afford many of the things other kids had, so I was always careful not to ask them for trivial items. But somehow, they managed to give us everything we needed. God has an amazing ability to stretch out the dollar.

I remember wanting to enroll in gymnastics classes so badly I could not help myself and asked my mom. I knew as soon as the words left my mouth it would not be possible.

"You want to take these classes because your friends are enrolled, Tiger. Is this right?" she asked while folding laundry, a never-ending chore in our busy family. On top of taking care of the four kids and my dad, she also worked in a local school as a daycare provider.

I felt guilty after asking her, and even more so because I was only a girl. She and my father had never intentionally made Loren or me feel less than our brothers, but we knew the Jordanian view on the place of girls in the family. I think that nagged at my mother as well because we are not from a family of complacent women.

She grew up with the same expectations for a woman in an Arab household and, like me, she had a strong mother who had chosen her own path. My mother had gone off to college to study in Beirut as a young woman, perhaps inspired by her own mother's courage to break with tradition and marry a man of her own choosing rather than a man selected by her parents. Both actions were seen as taboo in this rigid culture. My grandmother and mother were still dutiful wives—make no mistake about that.

In fact, Taita took the role of dutiful wife to new extremes. My grandmother was an incredible woman—smart, funny, a good wife, well respected in her village. She had the fewest kids in her community, a measly nine compared to the thirteen to fifteen most women had. Late in grandmother's pregnancy with my Aunt Ellen and she was hosting a dinner for some business acquaintances of my grandfather's. They had stopped by unexpectedly, but my grandmother was never caught unaware.

Without missing a step, she greeted them, served them beverages, and went into the kitchen to prepare dinner. While she was cooking, she went into labor and gave birth to my aunt by herself on the kitchen floor. Then, she matter-of-factly took little Ellen and bathed and swaddled her, all while making sure dinner was coming along properly. When dinner was ready, she served the food to her husband and his guests.

She was so calm that at first nothing out of the ordinary was noticed. But after doing a double-take, one of the guests asked, "Weren't you just pregnant?"

"Yes. I was, but I have given birth," she calmly replied, as though that wasn't any reason for alarm.

I like to imagine them just gawking at her, speechless.

So, when I asked my mother for gymnastics lessons, I thought of the generations of women's voices saying in her head, *You can do anything you put your mind to.*

Somehow my mother managed to get me those lessons. At the end of the day, we always got what we needed and never lacked any of the essentials. To this day, I still feel guilt within my gratefulness for the time I spent in gymnastics class. I have always wondered what it cost her.

But that voice was in my head as well. *You can do anything you put your mind to.*

School was more than just an opportunity for learning. More than an escape, it was now about maintaining my identity. I did not want to be Rinad the Cancer Patient. I wanted to be Rinad the Law Student.

I went in for a surgical biopsy to have one of the lymph nodes removed and discussed this dilemma with my surgeon. I think it is important to note that the surgeon was a female. I'd already heard the male perspective on my situation about chemo and law school. I was curious about a female perspective, especially someone in a field dominated by men who surely must have had her own challenges navigating gender expectations in our society.

When I told her what Dr. S had said about law school, she encouraged me to try.

"If you fail," she explained, "at least you will have given it your best effort and can look back with no regrets."

I took her advice and enrolled in my first semester.

CHAPTER 7

The Blackout

Five days before classes began, I got a port-a-cath (port, for short) surgically implanted into my chest for administering the chemotherapy drugs. Most forms of chemo are dispensed intravenously. Due to the caustic nature of the drugs, it is recommended that patients have this device inserted to maintain the integrity of the veins in their arms. After a few rounds of treatments, the veins start to collapse and it becomes nearly impossible to "find a good one" in order to administer the drugs. Ports are placed under the skin on the right side of the chest and are attached to a catheter that is threaded into a large vein above the right side of the heart called the superior vena cava. So, instead of fishing for a vein for every treatment or blood draw, the nurse just punctures the port site with a needle for easy access.

Some chemotherapy solutions are so corrosive that you will find sprinkler systems placed throughout chemo treatment rooms in case they spill all over someone because they will burn your skin off. Imagine that: something too toxic to touch that gets circulated through your veins.

After the port surgery, I went home and took a nap. When I woke up, I was drenched in sweat. I was sore where the port now poked out of my chest and still a little groggy from the anesthesia. My head hurt. I hadn't eaten, so I was also shaky.

Hysteria bubbled up like bile in my throat. Fleeing my bedroom, I discovered the air conditioner was off. I thought my father had turned down the air in an attempt to keep the electricity bill down, but it turned out there was a blackout covering all of New York.

I sank to the floor in the hallway, too emotionally exhausted even to walk back to my bedroom or seek out my parents. What had I done?

I was about to start law school *and* chemotherapy. Tackling even one of those things was enough to make most people nervous. I had signed up to do both at the same time. I had this horrible feeling in the pit of my stomach I had made the wrong decision. If I could barely survive the port insertion and a simple blackout without being hysterical, how would I survive the poison itself?

I also got incredibly angry at God. I'd been a good person up to this point in my life. Maybe not a saint, but I certainly didn't deserve this. Neither had my sister. Wasn't that in our contract with Him? Be a good person and He will shield you. I felt like He wasn't holding up His end of the bargain.

I was exhausted and sick and had not even begun classes yet. I had a foreign object sticking out of my bony chest that hurt every time I moved my arm. How would I get through this?

I thought of Aunt Ellen, the baby my grandmother had given birth to while cooking and serving dinner to a house full of guests. Aunt Ellen has played a major role in my life. She's been my guardian angel, my guiding light in times of distress when I felt lost and hopeless in the darkness. I don't know anybody who has worked as hard for anything in their life as Aunt Ellen. Her life was never easy.

At nine months old, Aunt Ellen had a high fever for several days, which made my grandmother nervous, so she took her to the village nurse. In a cruel twist of fate, the nurse used the same syringe he had used on someone who had polio to give my aunt a vitamin boost. My aunt contracted the disease and was left partially paralyzed. One leg became shorter than the other as she grew, and today she walks with a limp and has to wear a leg brace. She was told she would never have a normal life.

Under Jordanian standards, she would not be able to work, get married, or raise a family. Others believed she couldn't do what women were expected to do, and would have never been given an opportunity had she stayed.

Just as my mother had hoped, when she took Ellen with us to the United States, my aunt shined without the false boundaries of society. She enrolled in a renowned Christian university and worked full time to fund her education, a chance she never would have had in Jordan. Today, she has a PhD and leads a highly successful life, defying all those who believed she was broken and incapable. She has never let anybody tell her what she can or cannot do. She is vivacious and determined, and did not let her disability define her. She refused to be put into a box and have society place limitations on her.

When I was applying to college as a teenager, I wrote my admissions essays about how Aunt Ellen always inspired me to overcome obstacles. She was the most content person I knew because she never compared herself to anybody else. Had she succumbed to the temptation of comparison or viewed herself through the eyes of others, she may have started to see herself as limited by her disability and been unable to achieve the things she had. Her strong sense of self and surety in her value and worthiness made her the best role model I could have ever hoped for.

How could I do any less than meet this monster of chemo but head on? I could not start this challenge by feeling defeated. I wouldn't get past the first obstacle! In my head, I could hear the voices of the women in my family. *You can do anything you put your mind to.*

Finally, the day I came to dread arrived. My first chemo treatment. So much goes into preparation for chemotherapy it's exhausting. Chemotherapy is known to mess with the whole body. In fact, it is not doing its job unless it does.

Cancer is just a cluster of fast-growing cells, so chemotherapy is a toxic agent that kills all cells growing faster than normal. But guess what? Blood cells, skin cells, hair follicles, and digestive lining cells are also naturally occurring, fast-growing cells. In addition to killing off the cancer, chemo is programmed to attack and neutralize healthy cells that just happen to grow fast. That is why chemo patients experience nausea, hair loss, and skin flakiness and discoloration.

Before administering the chemo, the doctor checked my blood levels to make sure I could tolerate the chemo. White blood cells were checked because they are responsible for the body's immune system. Without a sufficient white blood cell count, my body could become *neutropenic* and unable to defend against foreign invaders such as viruses and bacteria. If my body's white blood cell count dipped too low, I would need an injection of Neulasta to stimulate the white blood cell growth. I would then need to have my blood retested in a few days to make sure my white blood cells were back to normal.

Another major blood test that must be done before chemotherapy is checking red blood cells because they are also affected by chemo. Red blood cells consist of hemoglobin, the iron-containing protein that transports oxygen from the lungs to other parts of the body. If my red blood cell count was too low, I would need a shot of Procrit to stimulate its growth.

The lab technician tested a host of other things as well and reviewed the results with the doctor. If all looked clear, I was sent up to the infusion room to get the pre-meds and ultimately the chemotherapy. The pre-meds often included Benadryl, in case of an allergic reaction, heavy steroids such as dexamethasone to calm any inflammation, and up to three different antinausea pills.

At this point, a numbing cream was applied to lessen the blow when the nurse stabbed the needle into my chest to gain access to the port. The nurse then "flushed the port" to make sure there was sufficient access to the vein and an adequate blood return. The vein had to be unobstructed; otherwise, the poison would linger around where it wasn't supposed to be. Saline, or sodium chloride, was used to flush the port, which in my case caused a metallic taste in my mouth. That sounds gross, but it has saved me so many times. If I didn't sense the metallic taste, then the vein was obstructed and the nurse needed to take the needle out and insert it again. Once the vein was open and operating, the chemotherapy drip could begin. These drips lasted four hours.

This seems like a lot, and it is, but after a while it's like clockwork.

My fear about making the wrong choice to tackle both chemo and law school only worsened the day after my first treatment. I questioned myself, wondering how on earth I could decide to take on chemotherapy and law school at the same time. I was nauseous, and I knew chemotherapy had a compounding effect—each future treatment would become more toxic. I also wondered if the stress of law school would exacerbate the cancer. But I put those fears to the back of my head. I didn't have room for all this negativity.

Classes started on a Monday and my chemotherapy was scheduled for every other Thursday for six months, in fourteen-day cycles. My constitutional equality law professor, Victor Goode, was one of the best teachers I have ever had. He meditated daily and knew the impact a healthy body had on maintaining a healthy mind. He told me whenever I was not feeling well that I could stay home and make up the work later.

I did not take advantage of this kind offer, wanting desperately to make a good impression. I also wasn't sure I could catch up if I ever got behind. But I appreciated the gesture.

I attended classes Monday to Wednesday, took Thursday off for chemo, and attended a morning class on Friday. Chemo hits the hardest on the third day, so by Saturday, I was feeling terrible. Sunday was spent recovering, and on Monday, I was back in class, doing it all over again.

During the second week of the cycle, the cumulative effect of the treatments began to take their toll. It was awful, but I could still function. I felt more myself by Thursday when the next treatment was scheduled. This happened twelve times in total: Tuesdays, sick with nausea and headache, every other Thursday, more chemo, recover . . . repeat. Two-thirds into the end of the treatment schedule, around the time of final exams, I was mentally and physically burnt out.

I learned that counting helped me cope when I would get nauseous. I would take deep breaths and count during the exhales until it subsided, almost like Lamaze. As the treatments continued, the counting got higher. It started with thirty, but after several weeks, we were in the triple digits. One night, I counted to three thousand before falling asleep, only to be woken twenty minutes later by another wave of nausea. I could not afford the luxury of cable TV, so I was at the mercy of regular network broadcasting. I would get a headache from all the static on each channel and found it was better to sit alone in the dark and wait it out. For days on end, I would sit alone in my room, waiting for the nausea to subside. Staring up at the ceiling, I tried to figure out how I got there.

I was allowed to take exams in a separate room. It wasn't so much for my convenience as it was for the other students. This way, I could take care of myself without disturbing them. I could eat or drink during the exam . . . or throw up. I remember vomiting several times during a torts exam. I kept running back and forth from the bathroom and I don't even remember actually finishing the test.

Throughout the semester, students volunteered to take notes for me on the days I couldn't make it to class. It is still incredible to me how much support I received from people who were, until then, complete strangers. I was able to handle all this stress because of people who stepped up even though they had never met me.

My new apartment in Queens was quaint and nothing fancy,

but I liked it. I could call it my own. Despite the treatment regimen I was bound to, I felt free again. I was fortunate to have found two very hospitable Iranian girls for roommates who treated me like family. They insisted I did not need to go home for chemo treatments but should stay in the apartment with them. They did not mind the constant flow of friends and family coming and going to take care of me.

When I look back at the situation now, I see the absurdity in it. I had just met these girls four days prior. I answered an ad at school stating a third roommate was needed. I met them that afternoon and signed the lease on the spot. Half a week later, I called them out of the blue to tell them I had just been diagnosed with cancer. I would think any other person would run for the hills or try to dissuade me from taking the apartment. But not these girls. From the first moment, they displayed love and support, offering me the same Middle Eastern hospitality my parents and grandparents had offered others over the years. This was just the beginning of the long list of people God would send my way to rally around and support me.

My parents were also supportive in so many ways. They brought me groceries and home-cooked meals. They did my laundry since there was no washer or dryer in my apartment complex and I didn't have the strength to haul it to a laundromat. They brought me snacks while I studied, prayed for me, and drove me to my appointments. My sister came to visit me on treatment weekends, which kept me from feeling alone, and I will always be grateful for that.

My older brother was incredibly supportive as well. When he found out about my diagnosis, he handed me his credit card and told me to use it liberally. He did not want me worrying about food or groceries and made it clear if I was ever too tired to take the bus to classes, I should call a cab on him. I tried not to take advantage of it—although I may have used it to buy a pair of shoes or two, purely for therapeutic purposes— but felt reassured that the option was there if I needed it.

I had the support system I'd seen rally around Loren when she fell ill. With everyone by my side, I started to feel like I could do this.

Many people ask me why I didn't stay home and defer school for a year when I was first diagnosed. It didn't occur to me to do that; it didn't occur to me to quit. When my sister was diagnosed, she stayed in college and finished out her senior year. She had two supportive roommates who got her through it. I knew I could do the same. I had my family. I had two incredibly compassionate roommates who became my family. We shopped and ate together, went to class and studied together. I really relied on them.

I looked forward to our evening tea and pound cake, where we would talk about our days. When I was in my twenties, I wanted my independence. Like my mother, I'd always kept my eye on what came next. I saw moving home as a step back.

I also thought I was supposed to learn from this experience. Up until now, every challenge had taught me important aspects of my character. Being the outsider in elementary school had started me on the path to discovering who I was as both a Jordanian daughter and an American woman. Rethinking medical school taught me that when something doesn't fit, I shouldn't try to force it; something better will come my way.

In my mind, it was starting to come together how good things can come out of bad situations, and that God is always in the middle of those storms. It was slowly becoming clear that just because I was suffering did not mean God had abandoned me. I was still blessed. People showed up for me and gave me love I felt I didn't deserve. I needed them and they were there, even though I didn't think I could give anything back.

I started to recognize a shift in my thoughts, which showed in the way I prayed and talked to God. I had started this difficult journey with a focus of, *Why are You doing this to me?* After just a short time, I'd transitioned to, *Okay, I'm not alone. I can do this.* It may not seem like a huge leap of faith, but for me, it was monumental. I was slowly learning that even though I may have gone to a lot of doctors' appointments and procedures on my own, I never felt alone. I'd always had my family around me to catch me if I stumbled, and I had God guiding my every step. However, it took a while for me to get out of the mindset of looking at life as "it's me against the world." I started slowly relying on others and on God for nearly every aspect of my daily survival. It was difficult for someone like me to live like that.

It was also extremely humbling.

From a very young age, we are taught about giving: by our parents, by our church, by the community at large. Cancer requires a self-centered obsession that overruled everything I had learned from my parents or my spiritual upbringing. It makes you selfish. Surviving takes every ounce of focus and strength to get through each day, and sometimes even that is not enough. There is nothing left to give back to others.

Without knowing it, however, I was giving back to my friends, and that's something that even now is helping me pay it forward. While in law school, my friends would take notes for me when I couldn't make it to class, which helped me stay caught up with my coursework. Part of my study routine was to make comprehensive outlines from everyone's notes, which I would then give back to my friends. Based on the work I did making those outlines, I later developed an iPhone app to help students study for the bar exam. It is available for free, and is called BARRED.

But it's hard to see the calm in the midst of a hurricane at times.

One of the most difficult storms I had to weather—and don't get me wrong, there are lots of side effects of cancer that are intolerable—was losing my hair.

I had what they called *beach waves*, the kind of long, dark, wash-and-go wavy hair that most girls dream about. Companies manufacture expensive saline solutions so girls with stringy hair can emulate the look.

When my hair started to fall out, it was heartbreaking. Wanting control of the situation, I had my sister take a razor to it, just as I had done for her years back. But the trauma soon had me in tears. And not the pretty tears that fall slowly down your cheeks. This was the heart-wrenching ugly cries that had me huddled on the bathroom floor while my sister cut away what remained of my hair.

It was another part of me, Rinad the Law Student, that I was losing to Rinad the Cancer Patient. It probably sounds vain or silly, but it goes back to my identity. I was working extremely hard to keep my life as normal as possible and this . . . this made it impossible not to see my life as anything but normal.

With every stroke of the razor, clumps would fall to the floor. With every lock of hair that fell to the floor, I felt less like myself. At least I had a chance of pretending I was healthy with a full head of hair. But as soon as you walk around bald, the secret is out. Everyone knows, and it is hard to avoid the big, bald elephant in the room.

CHAPTER 8

Don't Let the Cat
Out of the Bag

One of the most influential people I met during law school was Jeanne Anselmo, a registered nurse who specializes in holistic medicine. She instantly took me under her wing, and called me "Dear One." I knew instantly I was in good hands during that initial introduction. She told me about a new group called CUNY Contemplative Urban Law Practice (CCULP). They brought meditation and yoga classes to the students and faculty, and they thought I would be a good candidate for their services.

Joining that group taught me to stay centered during some of the hardest times at school. Jeanne was emotionally supportive and always helped me cope when it felt like the world was closing in. The perfectionist in me was still alive and well, and that meant making as few waves as possible in everyone else's lives. Yes, everyone was being helpful and supportive, but it caused me great anxiety to know that others were going out of their way for me. I can't explain why this caused me stress; it just did. I'd always worked toward my freedom, and even though I was living in my own apartment, I felt anything but free.

Jeanne introduced me to organic food, the importance of listening to my body, and above all, the value benefits of living in the moment. Jeanne later helped me find holistic treatments in lieu of the harsh regimen I had begun before school. She even set up a fund for me to spend on holistic remedies to counter the toxic effects of the chemotherapy, and I used the money to see a chiropractor and hypnotherapist.

I still needed to find a new oncologist, one close to school so I could continue my treatments without trekking all the way up to Westchester every other week. I found a C-rated doctor, Dr. K, close to my apartment in Queens. Since the chemo was standard protocol, I figured there was no harm in switching to a doctor who wasn't as highly recommended as Dr. S. Dr. K was hopeful and echoed what Dr. S had already told me, that even though any form of cancer is bad, Hodgkin's is the best kind to have, and I would be cured in six months.

I took this to heart. I was following the chemo protocol to the letter. While the toxins were taking their toll, I was restoring my body and mind with Jeanne's regimen of yoga and healthy eating.

A big challenge during this time was my parents' insistence against telling anybody about my illness. They were firm believers in not talking about negative things. *If you dwell on the negative, it becomes your reality*, they constantly reminded me. They did not want me to have to keep repeating all the dreadful details to well-meaning but curious friends and relatives. Rather than live in the misery of the illness, they wanted me to focus on the positives of law school and life in New York City. They wanted me to preserve whatever energy I had for healing by eliminating the negativity.

In Jordan, any kind of disease places a stigma on the whole family, and my parents didn't want me to live with that hanging over my head. I couldn't help but wonder if they worried it would hurt their prospect of making a good marriage match for me later on, and that is why they wanted to keep my illness a secret. If people knew I was ill, would they stop seeing me as a potential bride for their sons? I knew my parents had my best interests in mind, but it still made me question.

It took a few years to move past their insistence, to accept they were not ashamed of me. They wanted me to live, and in their minds, I had the best chance of surviving by focusing on the positive. It was their way of protecting me. Their culture understood things differently, and they reacted within the constraints of that understanding. As with so many other times in my life, the two sides of my upbringing clashed. I was again walking the line between the dutiful Jordanian daughter and the independent American girl.

In the end, I was the dutiful daughter and kept this secret to myself.

CHAPTER 9

She Made Me Soup

After the third chemo treatment, I started feeling some shortness of breath but waited to report it to my doctor. It progressively worsened until I could no longer climb a flight of stairs without gasping for air. At my fourth treatment session, I told the physician's assistant (PA). He looked at me with concern and told me I might have Bleomycin toxicity, but there was no way to confirm it without more testing.

We could not perform the tests that day because the doctor was not in the office and I was scheduled to have my treatment. It was important to stick to the schedule, he pressed. The PA gave me two choices: take the treatment as planned, which included the chance of damaging my lungs beyond repair, or skip the Bleomycin and risk the cancer persisting.

How could he expect me to make such a drastic life-altering decision on the spot like that? Up until then, I'd never had to make a choice harder than what I should major in or where I should go on spring break. How could I ever make an enormous decision like this and live with its eternal consequences?

I was angry at having to make that choice. I was twenty-three. I should be worried about what to wear for Saturday night dates, not about dire decisions that could irreparably damage my lungs and threaten my life. I thought of others my age, still living at home, not worrying about paying rent, spending their money on clothes and gadgets. I had to go to school, get passing grades, pay tuition. My biggest dilemma at this point should have been deciding where I was going to clerk that summer, not debating if I should stop a life-saving drug.

It was too much for anyone, let alone a twenty-three-year-old. And I was alone, I had no one to make this decision with me that day, not even my doctor.

So why wasn't another doctor paged? A change in treatment like that should include the weigh-in of a doctor, not just the physician's assistant. Feeling the ticking clock, and the pressure of the PA waiting for me to decide, I made a decision on the spot and chose to continue taking the Bleomycin.

In hindsight, it was the wrong choice, but I was still at the point of trusting the doctors and medical staff as authority figures on my disease. I wanted to follow the rules and get rid of the cancer. My goal posts had not changed.

My luck being what it was, both severe reactions happened; my right lung was eventually destroyed *and* the cancer persisted. Neither of us saw that coming. Like clockwork, my symptoms grew even worse after treatment. My breathing quickly deteriorated after that, and I had no choice but to stop taking the Bleomycin.

If there was a lesson to be gained from all of that, it was to take my time and follow my intuition. I should have demanded the necessary tests and put off the treatment for a few days, as my gut was demanding of me in that moment. I now believe this is one of God's ways of watching over us, like a gentle nudge in the right direction. For instance, I was in a lot of pain after one of my treatments and had a strange craving for cherries. At the time, cherries were not in season, but that didn't stop me from sending Loren on a wild goose chase all over town. She finally came back after an hour with a small bag of cherries that cost sixteen dollars! The following day, I read in a health magazine that cherries have medicinal properties that help ease pain. My body was telling me the solution without my brain consciously knowing it. And it didn't just happen once.

A few months later, during radiation therapy, I developed cravings for seaweed. The mere mention of seaweed sent my mouth watering. Luckily, I lived near Chinatown so finding dried seaweed was much easier than finding the cherries. I have always enjoyed sushi and foods that use seaweed ever since I believed I was Japanese, but these cravings were next level. I bought sheets of dried seaweed and ate it for snacks. I would pick up miso soup and take it back to my apartment and let the umami broth warm my chest. I later found out that miso soup and seaweed have health benefits for victims of radiation poisoning. Studies were conducted in Japan after the bombings of Hiroshima and Nagasaki during World War II.

Unfortunately, cherries and seaweed weren't enough to keep my nausea at bay. I was also taking Zofran, an anti-nausea medicine prescribed to patients receiving chemo and to pregnant women. It helped a little, but it was not enough. I thought since pregnant women took a certain dosage, I could double it and not harm myself. That was not the best idea. I became dizzy, developed a migraine, and vomited violently for days.

My sister took me to an urgent care facility after four days of these symptoms, and we found out that—no surprise—I had overdosed on Zofran. I was admitted to the hospital to have it cleared out of my system. To replace the Zofran, the doctor prescribed a synthesized medication that suppressed my central nervous system. I'm not sure which was worse. The new medicine was so debilitating that it left me unable to walk or move. One episode came at a particularly terrible time.

My family and friends had been a phenomenal source of support, but one afternoon, as fate would have it, everyone was out of touch. I was all alone in my apartment in Queens. I was hungry, but I was so drugged I could not walk to the kitchen for food. Not letting a little thing like the inability to walk get in my way, I rolled off my bed and crawled slowly to the kitchen. I wasn't strong enough to open the door to the fridge, so I lay there, motionless, for fifteen minutes until I gathered enough strength to crawl back to bed.

I then gave myself a pep talk, mustered all the strength I had, and crawled to the fridge once more . . . and again the door would not budge. After that, it took an hour to crawl back to bed. Believe it or not, I tried a third time. While I was lying helpless on the kitchen floor, the refrigerator door resolutely shut. I thought of various ways to get help. I could call my dad. *How would I open the door to let him in?* I couldn't even throw keys down to him through the window. That would require me to open a sliding glass door twice as heavy as the fridge door.

I had never felt more alone or more afraid than in those moments. I cried. I prayed. I cried some more. Anger welled inside at the unfairness of it all. I tried to channel the anger into something more productive, more Christian. *God never gives us more than we can bear.* I repeated that inside my head. Was crawling across the floor supposed to teach me humility? I rubbed my bald head. I thought I'd learned that lesson pretty well already. Was I supposed to remember that there was food available, even if I couldn't get to it? Not everyone had such luck.

The waves of self-pity started to recede, but I still felt pretty raw by the time my roommate Raha came home from class. She picked me up off the floor, helped me back to my bed, and made me some soup. In the end, I think this happened to remind me to be grateful because, for all the negative going on in my life, there was still plenty of positive. I had a safe place to live, food to eat, and family and friends to help. After that day, I developed a daily mantra: Any day I am well enough to feed myself is a good day.

Sure, I was fighting for my life. But I was not fighting alone. God made sure of that. My classmate Ajay then came into my life.

✝

Ajay was exactly the person I needed at that point. He played a tremendous role in helping me complete my second semester.

Ajay didn't know I had cancer at first. I heeded my parents' wishes and wore that pretty close to the vest around most people. Ajay and I hadn't gotten to know each other that well yet.

Since the treatments caused me to go bald, I wore a bandana that matched my sneakers. I thought it gave me a bit of a fashion edge, and it helped me feel less like the sick, bald girl.

One day while we were joking around, he started poking fun at me for wearing a bandana every day. "You look like Aunt Jemima."

I was embarrassed and a little angry and the words spilled out before I could think about it. "I have cancer. Hodgkin's Lymphoma Stage 3B. The chemo . . . well, I don't have any hair." I pulled the bandana from my head to show him.

His face transformed from gentle teasing to complete mortification. "I'm so sorry, Rinad. You totally rock the bandana look, hair or not." We both smiled as I put the bandana back on my head. "Seriously, if you ever need anything, I'm there, okay?"

And I believed him. The thing is, many people offer their help, but few ever come through with it. I could tell there was no falseness behind his words. Maybe people are right when they say that boys tease the girls they like.

I took him up on his offer, and he agreed to take me to my doctor's appointments and grocery store runs. I could always count on him. I was a little bird to nurture, and he reveled in the role of caretaker. We quickly became friends—then best friends.

We spent so much time together that eventually our feelings deepened. He was the epitome of generosity and kindness, and his soft-spoken nature attracted me. But most importantly, he was able to make me laugh.

He'd leave funny little doodles in the margins of notes he'd share from class, or send me a text of two pigeons fighting over a French fry in Central Park. Anything to get a smile out of me, especially on treatment days.

And that sealed the deal when he asked me out on a date. Of course, I said yes. Once we shifted our relationship from platonic to romantic, I came to rely on him even more. He wasn't just my best friend; he was my support. My boyfriend. I was no longer the freak cancer girl everyone pitied. Someone actually picked me and was public about it. I didn't have to spend my Saturday nights alone staring at the wall anymore.

I had someone *choosing* to be in the trenches with me.

CHAPTER 10

PET Tiger

My last treatment was at the end of January 2004. My mother came to the hospital to see me and brought me a stuffed tiger. As she handed it to me, she said she was proud of my strength and that I had graduated from a cat to a tiger. My parents and siblings were so happy that this ordeal was finally over. They were certain I was going to be cured just like my sister had been, and my father was already looking to the future, eagerly awaiting my graduation from law school.

But I am not my sister, and sometimes even when you play by the rules, life is not fair. You do not get the prize you thought you were promised.

Six weeks after my last treatment, a routine PET scan found a mass in my chest. A CT scan, then a biopsy, confirmed it was cancerous. This biopsy, called a mediastinoscopy, was far more invasive than the previous one. It involved cutting a huge slit across my throat and sticking a camera down with a needle on the end to collect a tissue sample. This left a one-inch scar across my neck, completely visible. My sister had a matching scar.

The mass sent shockwaves through my family and exposed the fragility of their confidence that all would be well. Immediately, everyone was in disaster mode, frantically searching for the next step to restore normalcy. The oncologist referred me to a radiation therapist who recommended a treatment plan that included blasting my neck, chest, and back with high doses of radiation.

I was immediately against it because of the risk of radiation causing more cancer and further damage. So, I looked into alternative therapies. I'd already learned this lesson from the incident with the Bleomycin toxicity.

Listen to your intuition, Rinad, my inner voice was saying. *God is trying to lead you somewhere.*

My family was in an uproar. They couldn't understand the concept of rejecting a doctor-prescribed treatment. My mother said I had already been through the worst, so I should just follow through and get it over with. My father agreed, adding that radiation was not as hard as chemotherapy. I wish that were true.

But it's difficult to ignore the advice of your parents, the two people you know will protect you against all things.

Follow the rules.

Get the prize.

I had followed the rules with my initial diagnosis. I had followed the same path Loren had taken after her own diagnosis. Only our paths were now diverging.

Hesitantly, my radiation oncologist referred me to a specialist for a second opinion at a world-renowned facility that only treats cancer. This new doctor only increased the recommended treatment, stating that since the cancer originally stretched from my neck down to my stomach, they should radiate the entire field.

I would later learn the real reason for this more aggressive recommendation—funding at these facilities depends on the patients' initial survival rates. If they kept the patients alive—not necessarily thriving, but alive—they would get their money. Therefore, cancer specialty centers invariably overmedicate to ensure their patients survive, even if it contributes to long-term problems.

Because of this, I advise newly diagnosed patients to get a second opinion from a non-cancer center whose funding doesn't rely on numbers and ranking.

Since I wasn't strong enough to ignore my doctor's recommendation for radiation, back I went to the hospital to begin the prescribed treatment: five days a week for six weeks.

Once again, I was going to follow the rules, even though my intuition was screaming at me to break free. I don't put any blame for my decision on anyone. I listened to the doctors. I made my decision. It's hard to go against the advice of doctors when you're facing a life-or-death choice. You're convinced they want you to live as much as you want to live. Why be a doctor if not to save people? I've since learned there's a big difference between saving people and practicing medicine.

It would have been impossible to continue classes on my own, but Ajay stepped up to meet my needs. He drove me to and from my appointments every day and made the situation bearable. I would have never gotten through that semester without him.

My overwhelming need for Ajay's support also made it easy to ignore the bigger issues in our relationship while I was sick. As my health improved, it was harder to put those problems aside.

I'd always been very open about my desire to marry a Christian man, and since Ajay was not one, we could never take our relationship to the next level. He resented the Christian dominance and historical colonization of non-Christian cultures and saw my hard line as an example of that. Perhaps it was just selfishness on my part, another example of the fear cancer had put inside of me that I would not get what I wanted out of life. I felt I had to work harder to fit what life I did have into the mold I'd created, and Ajay was bearing the brunt of that. But in the end, I wanted to marry a Christian man, so I told Ajay our relationship would never evolve because he wasn't one. We were not meant to be. Months later, after a year and a half of sharing this journey, we parted ways.

I am pleased to report that Ajay went on to find happiness with someone who shared his goals and beliefs. I will always be grateful for the role he played in my life. He set the bar so high for what I should expect in a life partner, a bar no one was able to reach for almost fifteen years. It would take that long for me to be vulnerable with someone again.

At the time, however, it didn't take me long to realize how hard it would be without Ajay in my life. Two weeks after our breakup, I was out of remission and facing yet more rounds of chemo and radiation.

Only this time I would be facing them without Ajay to help.

†

Life during radiation treatment was a waking nightmare. The radiation caused third-degree burns on my chest and upper back. Layers of skin would peel off with my clothes, so I was forced to wear camisoles that exposed the affected area. Even uncovered, the pain was excruciating. It grossed out my classmates, one of whom wasn't too shy to let me know.

While waiting for class to start one day, one of the other students actually approached me and said, "I know you're sick, but could you maybe wear a jacket or just not come to class until you're healed? It's a little unnerving seeing your raw flesh exposed."

My mother was right: Bisseh was no more. I had graduated to the tiger. I went to class anyway. I had no choice. I pushed on, and I got through my courses and my treatments.

The bright side of radiation, if you can find one, was that I did not experience the nausea or hair loss the chemo presented. In fact, my hair was starting to grow back in. I was able to get rid of the bandanas and let my hair grow naturally. My best friend came down from Philly to pamper me on a Manhattan weekend getaway. We booked two nights in the Plaza Hotel, went to a trendy restaurant for dinner, treated ourselves to matching haircuts at the highly sought-after Frédéric Fekkai salon, and she topped off the weekend surprising me with a heart-shaped necklace from Tiffany's to hide my scar. It was exactly what I needed after such an atrocious year. But unfortunately, life didn't get easier after radiation.

To my horror, my post-radiation PET scan did not show clean margins.

Adding to the nightmare, Dr. K dumped me as a patient, although this should not have come as a surprise; he was not supportive during my chemotherapy treatments. His reasoning for passing me off was that, because my scans didn't come back clean, I'd likely need a bone marrow transplant, which he couldn't administer. He referred me to a specialist in the Bronx to confirm. I didn't trust Dr. K's judgment by this point, so I also made an appointment to get a second opinion at a renowned facility in Manhattan.

Another biopsy would be needed to confirm the mass in my chest was in fact cancer, but before even doing so, the Manhattan doctor called all of my family in for blood samples to see if any of them were a match for a transplant. Something about that didn't sit right in my stomach, but I let it go initially. This doctor explained her hastiness by saying that the success of cancer treatment is dependent on timing, and insurance companies can be notorious for taking their sweet time approving procedures.

However, before confirming I even needed the transplant, the same doctor scheduled me for an appointment to begin harvesting bone marrow. No biopsy had been performed yet! They didn't even know whether I needed a transplant and wanted to perform a painful and invasive procedure *just in case.*

The truth was, the Manhattan hospital had "open bed syndrome." Their transplant ward was empty and they needed patients and were prepared to prescribe a bone marrow transplant whether I needed one or not.

I declined their offer.

Luckily, Dr. K came through in one area for me: his referral to the Bronx specialist, Dr. W. He had the opposite approach. He did not want to rush into a bone marrow transplant and instead monitored me for a year before prescribing a course of treatment.

Throughout this year of observation, I was on constant pins and needles. Every successive scan showed some areas with masses spreading and others where they were disappearing. To track the ever-changing landscape of the alleged cancer, I got a PET scan every month from May 2004 until February 2005.

The word *PET* sounds approachable, cute even, something you could look forward to. It isn't. It's actually rather hazardous. A PET scan is a nuclear imaging scan using radionuclides, also known as tracers, made of radioactive liquid glucose.

First, the patient is starved for twelve hours, then injected with the tracers. The starving body eats the radioactive glucose, and the cells that eat the fastest are the cancer cells. They appear darker in color as they eat more of the glucose solution. The PET scan captures the image of where the tracers are and where they are traveling. Next, a large X-ray machine is used to photograph the body to look for the darker cancerous cells.

Doing this exposes the body to a high amount of radiation. Patients are literally radioactive for twenty-four hours after the test. Because of this, they have to be quarantined until it's safe for them to come into contact with other people. When patients are discharged, they are given a doctor's note in case they trip the alarm on a metal or radiation detector. It's more common than you might think.

I don't like thinking about all the toxicity pumped through my body in those nine months and the years that followed. After February 2005, I had a PET scan every three months for the next four years, then yearly for a period. I am now back to going every six months. This test will always be a part of my life, and it makes me anxious thinking about the long-term side effects all of that radioactivity and radiation will have on me. The sad truth is, if the cancer doesn't kill you, the testing and treatments might.

Dr. W had been in the cancer business a long time, and even with his vast experience, he had never seen Hodgkin's behave this way—spots visible on one scan but gone the next. Every successive scan showed some areas with masses spreading and others where they were disappearing. Dr. W became convinced this wasn't cancer.

"Untreated," he told me one afternoon while reviewing my scans, "cancer always gets worse, never better." Under normal conditions, untreated aggressive cancer would have killed me within a year. I was still alive and kicking. Because the PET scan showed visible changes each month, Dr. W thought it was inflammation rather than cancer. The problem, however, is you can't test for inflammation. It's simply wait and see.

I was in limbo, a state of being I would quickly get used to. But I liked this doctor and respected him. It is rare for me to say that about doctors, but I felt like this one actually cared about me, not my numbers; he didn't want to keep me alive only so he could tout his success rate. He actually cared about my well-being. He always treated me with extra care. It may have been because I was fifty years younger than his other patients, or maybe I reminded him of his granddaughter, but he always gave me special attention. He answered my calls immediately, gave me my own private room during transfusions, and squirreled away treats for me left behind by the pharma reps.

Small gestures go a long way, and there are no small kindnesses when you are fighting for your life. Dr. W didn't just treat my cancer; he treated *me*.

I liked his laid-back approach. He wasn't the type of doctor who went into situations with guns blazing. He was more conservative with his treatment protocols, and that made me appreciate him more.

Then one month, his prognosis was tested. My red blood count was low and he feared that if I did have cancer, it may have spread to my bones. His prescription was to eat meat three times a day for a month. If my red blood cells went up, it was anemia, not cancer. I returned the next month to find that organic red meat had saved me from a very painful bone marrow biopsy.

But as we waited, I developed a very strange symptom. Every time

I drank red wine, even a small sip, I got shooting pains in my hip and lower back, the same areas where the new masses were showing up on the scans. This time, Dr. W changed his diagnosis. He now believed it was cancer, citing another rare symptom of Hodgkin's Lymphoma—besides the excessive itching where you feel you want to peel your skin off, like Loren had suffered—experiencing pain when certain vices are ingested, such as wine or other kinds of alcohol.

He ordered an X-ray guided biopsy, but the mass didn't show up on the screen. That should have been enough for him to stop, but instead, he ordered a surgical biopsy. A surgeon then slit my thigh open, tore through the muscle, and drilled a hole in my hip. He was convinced there was a tumor and would not stop until he found it.

He did not find a tumor. To this day, I still have a nasty scar and can't sit with my legs folded, even though the biopsy was performed sixteen years ago.

The biopsy report came back showing the bone was benign and I was officially in remission for the first time, one year and six months after my initial diagnoses. Although I was on crutches for a few weeks and used a cane for several months, all that mattered was I was in remission.

That was how I celebrated Valentine's Day 2005, recuperating in a hospital bed. Finally, my ordeal was over. I'd followed the rules. I was in remission. That was what I focused on. As long as I avoided red wine, I was perfectly healthy.

I could loosen the noose around my neck and begin to enjoy life again. My first year of law school was wrapping up. I had finished with honors and was determined to graduate with my classmates. I made plans with friends, traveled a little, and tried to enjoy the summer before school started up again in the fall.

Things had finally started looking up, or so I hoped.

Life #2

CHAPTER 11

Who's the Ghost Now?

That summer was as much a celebration as it was a time of recuperation. My body had been through hell. As hard as I tried to show a tough demeanor, my mind and heart had not escaped the torment unscathed. I turned to my faith, to prayer to help ease the doubt that was a constantly nagging voice, egged on by fear and uncertainty.

Despite all that, I still enjoyed the summer as best I could. I lived with my parents up in Westchester and clerked at the same law firm I had worked in the previous summer. I had done some non-legal related work with this law firm before I started law school, and out of the blue, the managing partner called me and asked if I wanted to summer clerk with his firm before I started law school.

I jumped at the opportunity to get the experience under my belt and on my resume. It was well known that the firm you "summer" with most likely becomes the firm you get an offer with after graduation, and this was one of the more reputable firms in Westchester County. I also enrolled in criminal procedure and commuted to Queens twice a week to make up some credits.

Professionally, it was an exceptionally good time for me, but I was very busy.

In the rare quiet moments when I found myself alone, my mind wandered again and again to my faith and my connection to God. In many ways, I was at a high point in my faith. Yes, I had struggled and doubted. I had even ignored God's voice through my intuition. But I'd made it. I'd followed the rules as a Christian—prayer, belief, faith—and I was rewarded. Whatever trials or failures I'd endured with my faith, I must have made up for them because God had seen me through.

I knew I wasn't out of the woods. If there'd been an obscure, long-term side effect of a drug or treatment plan, I seemed to have found it.

But it's amazing how easily we fall back into old habits once there's a calm in the storm.

However, the silver lining on the cloudy days of the previous eighteen months didn't last long. The Fourth of July weekend arrived, and it brought with it anything but independence.

I was in Boston for the holiday when the recognizable signs of sickness poked holes in my calm facade. It started with a cough, and the familiar hacking made me pause. When it didn't go away after several weeks, I went to see my oncologist. He did all the various tests, and my worst fear was confirmed.

The cancer had come back.

✝

Dr. W believed I should begin a cocktail of MVP (Mitomycin-C, Vinblastine, Cis-Platin) right away. Although this was not the FDA-approved chemotherapy treatment plan for relapse patients, he believed I had the best shot of kicking it for good with this concoction as opposed to the bone marrow transplant. I would learn later that this doctor was way ahead of the curve on treatment protocols.

But MVP was not without risks. He warned me the cocktail would wreak havoc on my bone marrow and white and red blood cells. I would be more immunosuppressed and would have to spend weeks in isolation after treatment because of the risk of infection. I would also become anemic and would need daily Procrit shots to stimulate red blood cell development and would have to administer these shots myself. In addition, I would also need blood transfusions, *and* the Vinblastine would likely collapse my veins since I was adamant against getting another port. It was uncomfortable because it sat right underneath my bra strap, and I could not move my arm without it rubbing up against the protrusion. I was always on the skinnier side and did not have the added cushion for protection.

I was deflated. I had been through so much already and every previous round of treatment had come with the promise of success. I did not want to go through any more chemotherapy. It had not worked before and arguably made my situation worse. How could putting more poison into my body be the answer?

It can't be the only answer, my instinct was telling me. I liked and trusted Dr. W, but I did not like the news he was delivering. Talk about shooting the messenger. *This was one doctor's opinion,* I told myself. Surely there had to be others. Was this another nudge from God that I needed to listen to? I wasn't going to ignore my intuition this time.

I went in search of another option. I researched various clinics and holistic therapies. I looked into a clinic in Texas, but they only worked with brain tumors on children. I found a clinic in New York and made an appointment to see them; however, the first topic of discussion was payment. They would not even give a consultation without receiving compensation upfront. The bill for the consultation alone was $250, and the cost of services would likely have been in the ballpark of $20,000 for a regimen of supplements over six months.

Every day, I found another dead end. Listening to my intuition was not easy because every dead end put my family more on the edge, pleading with me to reconsider the chemo.

My sister, in particular, begged me to start treatment. "Time is crucial, Rinad," she told me over the phone one evening when I'd called to discuss a holistic treatment center in Mexico. I trusted her opinion because she'd been where I was, at least in part. Her treatments had been successful, but she knew the pain and disruption chemo had on your life. "You cannot take any chances with feel-good, New Age wannabe doctors that just want to take you for every penny."

We had been raised together and had heard our parents exclaim many times over the power of prayer. Prayer and faith had led our mother from her home in Jordan to the United States. Faith in a Higher Power had kept our family going during lean times, when money was scarce. Prayer had played a significant role in our family during her own fight against cancer. We'd always believed God would bring us to a better place by answering our prayers.

Would she understand this feeling I had, this intuition that God's voice was trying to lead me somewhere different?

When I think back to our childhood or the many things she and I had shared as young women with so much in common, we'd never talked about our faith. Like many things in our lives—education, the acceptance of a daughter's place in a Jordanian household, introductions to a future husband—we simply accepted what we were given. Our faith and our religious beliefs were as much a part of our cultural heritage as our language or marriage choices.

In the end, I kept my beliefs about my intuition and God's voice to myself because I did not want to go against the grain. *Surely if God was speaking to me, He would have the same message for my parents as well*, I rationalized. The logical part of my brain could hear the words, and even I rolled my eyes a little. *God's voice*, I laughed at myself. *Why would God be talking to me? He's put doctors and proven treatments in front of you, Rinad. Don't be ridiculous.*

I hate to admit it, but I gave in to my family's rational arguments. Honestly, I didn't have the money to pay for the natural, holistic treatments, though I like to think I could have found a way; I always did. I chose traditional Western medicine once again, even though the very essence of who I was—Bisseh—was telling me to fight against tradition and pick my own path.

As advertised, the MVP treatments roasted my bone marrow and turned my body into a war zone. My white and red blood cells retreated like Napoleon from Moscow after the first treatment, and it was already time for reinforcements in the form of my first red blood transfusion.

I was freaked out.

The thought of receiving someone else's blood was something reserved for really sick people —the last hope of the dying. Even with everything going on, I didn't see myself that way. Sure, I was sick; I was Rinad the Cancer Patient, but I wasn't Rinad the *Dying* Cancer Patient. I was getting cured.

In the end, I had no choice. It may all be a numbers game for hospitals looking at funding, but it's also a numbers game for patients' survival, and my numbers were telling me to accept the transfusion. When I did, the results left me amazed! I immediately felt better. It was like I had been starved and then given my favorite food.

I had more color in my cheeks—the usual rosiness I had, like the midwife described when I was born, returned. It was a rebirth. I had more energy; I felt alive. It was instantaneous. I came to depend on the transfusions, needing two or three a month, to keep me bouncing back enough to keep moving forward.

But there were days during the treatment when I didn't think I could open my eyes or get out of bed. A wave of dizziness could hit me like a random thought while I was walking down the street, so strong

I had to stop and hopefully find a place to sit down until it passed. My blood pressure went up and down, and my heart, already showing signs of stress from the Adriamycin during my first treatment plan, would race uncontrollably at times.

It finally hit me—I was that dying person. What a harrowing revelation. It changes you on a fundamental level. You see yourself both as incredibly strong for making it through the ordeal, but also incredibly weak, knowing the war raging in your body.

I experienced severe panic attacks, a first for me. I'd never dealt with more than the usual anxiety in life at high-stress moments: waiting for my acceptance to George Washington, waiting to hear about the results of the LSAT or my application to law school. Much like my nickname, Bisseh, I'd sit back and observe until I pounced. Once my back was up, however, watch out.

But this was different. I wasn't in charge... of anything. My treatments were the purview of the doctors. The schedule was determined by assistants and nurses. Some days I could barely feed myself or get up to take a shower. I relied on my generous family and support group of friends to put food on the table, make sure I had clean clothes, or pick up my medicines when needed. Cancer is selfish. It was more in charge of my life than I was.

On New Year's Eve, I was dining with friends in a crowded French restaurant. It was a rare day when the treatments and recovery periods had aligned and I was feeling almost human again. The din of conversation around the table would normally be background noise, but today it echoed in my head. My friends were laughing and joking, talking about the useless, miscellaneous stuff that fills up our days and lives when you don't have to fight cancer and can just jump out of bed to face the day.

I was almost scared to eat the soup I'd ordered, worried it would upset my stomach, but I took a few gentle sips anyway, trying for any semblance of normalcy. The rich aroma of their cassoulet and coq au vin wafted around the table, foods I wanted to try, but I knew my stomach couldn't handle the rich, heavy dishes.

Then I saw him.

Staring.

Under usual circumstances, a handsome man staring at me would send my heart racing. But when he caught me looking, he quickly looked away, and the pity on his face let me know he wasn't attracted to me. I ran my hand over my hair, thin as it was. I'd taken pains with my appearance, putting on makeup and wearing my favorite little black dress and heels. It was an outfit that normally garnered quite a different reaction from men.

The walls started to close in on a wave of heat, and an impending sense of doom flared hot and fast. *Am I seriously having a hot flash right now?* My brain started to race, but it would fast-forward, then slam on the brakes. The room tunneled to a distant pinpoint of light, the voices of my friends and the people around me disappearing down the long, dark void.

Breathe, Rinad. Breathe. I coached my lungs as they began to close, my fingers pressing into the edge of the table. My legs were shaking now, so I counted. *One, two, three. . . .*

This is not me, I convinced my brain and my arms and legs and any other parts I thought might listen. I wasn't going to fall apart in the middle of dinner in a fancy French restaurant. But just like trying to convince myself not to have cancer didn't work, convincing myself not to fall apart didn't work either.

I pushed awkwardly from the table, all conversation suddenly halting mid-syllable as I felt the blood rush from my face to pool in my feet. I ran from the dining room, guided by blind luck and desperation, until I found the ladies' room. I pushed inside a stall, locked the door, and collapsed to the floor.

I didn't want this life. I didn't want a life of cancer treatments and blood transfusions and picking out wigs to cover my balding head when my hair fell out. I wanted casual conversations. I wanted my biggest worry to be where I would intern that summer.

This isn't fair! I screamed silently at God, the Universe . . . basically anyone who might be listening. *Why is this happening to me? This isn't what I was promised. Work hard. Study. Follow the rules.*

At twenty-five, I was completely overwhelmed by my life.

Somewhere along the way, my friends found me and called my sister. I rang in the new year curled up on the bathroom floor, waiting for her to rescue me.

The MVP treatment was absolutely awful. One of the bags they administered during each four-hour treatment was bright blue, and to this day, I can't drink anything blue without vomiting. My veins collapsed and hardened, just as predicted, due to the Vincristine. It became next to impossible to draw blood or administer IV fluids.

But that was nothing compared to the immunosuppression. After each treatment, I was required to be in isolation for two weeks and could not travel more than twenty miles from the hospital. If I spiked a fever, I could become septic, meaning my blood would become poisonous. If I didn't receive a full spectrum of antibiotics within six hours of a spike, I would die. Before I began the treatment, I had booked a yoga retreat with Jeanne, but I had to cancel, as the lodging was about forty miles away.

That wasn't the only thing to get canceled.

The restrictions of isolation after every treatment made attending classes impossible, so I was forced to drop the next semester in favor of trying to restore my health. I spent most of the treatment schedule living at my parents' house so they could take care of me. My brother, Tariq, stepped in again and offered to cover my rent, since I was not eligible for financial aid that semester. It was a relief, since I don't think I could have handled the stress of moving on top of all the other changes going on in my life.

In addition to the physical symptoms, I had a myriad of emotional and psychological roller coasters to ride during all of this. How anyone tolerated me is a testament to their patience, friendship, and love because I was almost painful to be around. I was irritable. I was angry. I became a pro at turning every conversation around to end with me having cancer and how much I hated it.

My emotional state was strangled by the word *unfair*. Why did I have to go through all of this? Why did I have to worry about PET scans and hair loss on top of final exams? When I look back, I can only shake my head at the powder keg on which my life perched. Law school alone is a lot of pressure. Dealing with cancer would be enough to put most on edge emotionally. Doing both at the same time? In a word . . . insanity!

I felt brittle. A strong wind would snap me in two. This was not a state I would have ever thought possible for Bisseh, the rosy-cheeked girl so full of life at birth. I wanted to be strong, to once more surpass all expectations and show the world what I was made of.

But I had little to nothing left to give.

Needless to say, I was definitely not an easy person to be in a relationship with, and truthfully, that's probably why Ajay and I broke up. I don't blame him for ending it; I didn't even want to be around me. I hated being in my own skin. On top of that, I was a second-year law student so that meant I knew everything. And even though I was always right, I had to argue with you to prove to you why I was. It's inevitable for a law student; a rite of passage. Suffice to say, it was a very lonely and miserable time in my life.

Some of that loneliness was self-induced, but I turned back to the things I had learned from my friend Jeanne and CCULP. Since I was unable to pursue a guided holistic program during this time, I decided to create my own. In the short window of days between each isolation period, I began taking multiple yoga classes, practiced daily morning meditation and visualization exercises, and attended intense psychotherapy, hypnosis, and weekly chiropractic sessions. I also implemented an all-vegan diet.

At this point, I desperately needed an escape from the ongoing mess my life had become, and since I had taken the semester off from school, I had too much time on my hands. I joined eHarmony. It was the perfect place to hide. I could be whoever I wanted to be: Rinad the Sexy Law Student rather than Rinad the Miserable Cancer Patient.

Every decision I was making in my life was made because of the cancer. It was always something in the back of my mind. Since breaking up with Ajay, the loneliness had gotten worse. I was still looking for my *person*, that one person to share my life, however long I had.

I went out on a lot of dates, but I never discussed my health issues. I didn't realize I was not ready for a serious commitment because I was not whole in body or spirit. I still didn't know who I was. Law student. Cancer patient. Dutiful daughter. Independent woman. How could I be the other half of someone if I didn't know who I was?

During that time, if I wasn't in the hospital or practicing my self-guided holistic treatment, I was out on dates. Sometimes four dates a week—including double-header Sundays where I had a brunch date in the morning and then a dinner date that same evening, trying to find an escape. For a couple of hours a week, I was able to fake a smile before reality collapsed on me.

It was great while it lasted, but like most periods of reprieve, it would soon turn sour.

I would meet a man on a date and there would be great chemistry.

We would go out two or three times, but invariably it would end because I would fake being whole and healthy, putting on a persona that was not the real me. They likely sensed I was hiding something—I was, after all—and it would all fall down like a house of cards.

So, the next time I tried something new: I wanted to be honest for a change. I met a guy named Jake who lived up in White Plains. He was an all-American guy—not something I was ever into before, but I was trying new things. We had a great time dating. It lasted about two months, just long enough for me to begin feeling comfortable around him. One night, against my better judgment, I told him I had cancer at the end of one of our dates.

I texted him to let him know I arrived safely, which was our usual ritual, but he didn't respond. The next day, same thing. My dating-senses were tingling. Loren, who always gave everyone the benefit of the doubt, believed he was lying somewhere in a ditch and I should at least call to make sure he was still alive. She was adamant he wouldn't *ghost* me.

I called him, and I could tell he was blowing me off because he sent me directly to voicemail. I was thinking, *Wow, he finds out I have cancer and might die, but he's the one who turns into the ghost.* Finally—normal twenty-five-year-old girl problems!

I canceled my eHarmony account that weekend.

It really sank in why my parents wanted to keep my illness a secret. People react one of two ways when you tell them you have a disease like cancer: they become supportive or they run in fear.

And believe me, I get the fear. I can't count the number of times I've wanted to run away from this diagnosis over the last eighteen years. Run far and run fast. Facing your own mortality is frightening, perhaps more so when you're in your twenties. But I'm stuck with it, and when people do react in fear, as if I'm contagious, it becomes a side effect of the disease for which there is no treatment.

I reminded myself I did not have time for these cowards. I had law school waiting and extra classes to make up for the missed semester. My life was tough enough, and I didn't need to make it worse pining after people who did not deserve to be a part of it.

Besides, I had been neglecting another relationship, and *it* was about to crash into me like a tidal wave.

CHAPTER 12

The Furry-Tailed Squirrel

On top of all my intensive holistic routines, I prayed like never before. If the breakdown in the bathroom on New Year's had shown me anything, it was that my relationship with God needed as much work as my health. Up until this point in my life, prayer had been about asking God for things. *Give me a cure. Let me live.*

Don't let me die.

Sitting on the cold floor in that bathroom, feeling as alone as I'd ever felt in my life, I kept asking, *Why me?* But something clicked while I waited for Loren. "Why me?" was as good a question as "Why not me?"

I tried a new tactic in my conversations with God.

Help me understand.

I believed the alternative approaches to traditional medicine—the yoga, the psychotherapy, the meditation—were expediting the healing process for my body and protecting me from the harsh side effects of the chemical cocktail being administered. Thus, I began to look for alternative healing approaches for my spiritual body. I needed help to understand what God wanted from me with this journey. If I could understand what I was supposed to learn, maybe the spiritual healing would precipitate the physical healing.

I started this healing by looking to my faith. That's not to say I didn't have faith, but my faith was blind; it was built on an acceptance of what I had been given as a child and not on anything I had cultivated and nurtured as an adult. In simpler terms, I had not yet earned my spiritual stripes. I was still a child when it came to my faith.

My relationship with God, in many ways, followed the same path as my diagnosis. I got sick, but even then, I figured I'd be better in a year. That was the journey I witnessed in Loren so that was the journey I expected to follow.

In much the same way, my parents had experienced difficult times. I never saw them change the way they expressed their faith or even display any doubt that this faith would be rewarded. Things always worked out for them by doing what they'd always done in the past.

I never felt the need to pray differently or explore my faith to a deeper degree. Mine was a social contract with God. I was a good person, so God would reward me, not rain terror on me. We had an understanding.

Until we didn't.

I never stopped believing in God during my journey to find a cure. And at first, I didn't think I really had a reason to be praying to a *Higher Power*. I was following the rules and thought I would be cured just like my sister, so why worry? Why appeal to some invisible being in the sky? I think I just saw Him as some entity who didn't seem to have much to do with me or the billions of others suffering down here on this chaotic orb.

But with each grueling day, as my cancer spread, my treatments got progressively tougher, and my health deteriorated, I began to wonder if I was doing something wrong. If He existed, and was ultimately in control, then reason could only lead me to believe He was *allowing* me to suffer. I was having a hard time justifying that He loved me *and* was allowing this to happen to me. I knew I was supposed to love God, but at this point, I mostly questioned Him. *What are you thinking?* I found myself asking. A lot. Healing that relationship would literally take an act of God!

This chemo cocktail was much worse than the previous treatments. The nausea, heartburn, and dizziness were overwhelming, and I wanted to quit many times, but my mom and sister kept me going. The familiar mantra *follow the rules, get the prize* was used as the carrot at the end of a stick.

One bright spot did make itself known, however. During the initial treatment of ABVD, I was told I had an 80 percent probability of losing my hair. I lost it all immediately. This time, the doctor said I had a 100 percent probability of losing my hair after the first MVP treatment.

I decided it would be less traumatizing to preemptively cut my hair. If it was short and falling out, it would not scar me as much as if it was long. Oh, the stories we tell ourselves. . . .

Loren and I were in the hair salon on a Saturday, one of its busiest days, with a customer at every station, stylists running between those customers, and others getting Brazilian blowouts or color highlighted around the perimeter like plastic-covered casserole dishes still warming in the oven.

I was on the chair in the hair salon, crying as the stylist made the initial chops to my longish hair. My sister, who is incapable of seeing someone cry alone, was sobbing too.

The poor hairdresser, holding a lock of my hair in her fingers, looked at us in the mirror, fear brightening her eyes. "Do you want me to stop?" She dropped the lock of hair as if it were a snake about to bite her, then hid the scissors behind her back.

"No," I sobbed. "It's going to fall out in a week or two. I might as well get the process started." I'd never come close to telling many friends or family about my health, and here I was telling a complete stranger.

The hairdresser nodded knowingly and the first tears shimmered on her lower lashes. "My mom," she choked out. Then without a word, she lifted the scissors and with three quick whacks, chopped off the ponytail riding at her neck.

My jaw dropped. Things around us started to go still in the bustling salon. The stylist to our right asked if everything was ok, and my hairdresser just nodded.

"Some things shouldn't be done alone," she said, dropping her hair to the floor to join mine. I watched the silvery-blonde wisps fall like snowflakes atop my darker brunette strands. "I've been wanting to donate it anyway."

When I looked back up, the hairdresser was leaning over my shoulder. "How about we go with a bob? I think we can both carry that off."

Still in shock at her action, I just sat there frozen. Loren started to laugh first, and was soon joined by a few other customers. Before I knew it, the entire shop was giggling. More importantly, I'd stopped crying.

I met the hairdresser's eyes in the mirror. "A bob."

This stranger's gesture filled me, like cool water over a parched desert, and I like to think it was God's voice in her actions answering my prayer, *help me understand*. I wasn't alone. I didn't know what had happened with her mom; I could guess. But I did know that like her, I wasn't walking alone. Others had walked my path before, and maybe one day I would be the voice that let people know they were not alone regardless of how lonely they felt, as their world crumbled.

Sometimes that's all you get. Sometimes that's all you need.

Having explored a variety of holistic and alternative healing methods, I'd come across a licensed hypnotherapist who'd worked with other cancer patients to lessen the side effects of chemo. She didn't promise cures. If she had, I doubt I would have believed anything she said. I really had nothing to lose—except my hair—and I didn't want to let the opportunity pass me by if this could make a difference. I added her to my alternative treatment plan and went to hypnosis to prevent the hair loss.

During our session, she told me to close my eyes and imagine a furry-tailed squirrel running circles in the yard. She wanted me to use my will and determination to keep my hair on my head. I won't say I wasn't skeptical, but it wouldn't be the first time I'd used sheer will to get something I wanted.

As a kid, I played with a little girl who lived up the street. I liked the little girl okay, but my interest in her was mainly for her baby brother, Danny, whom I wanted to pick up and hold. The little girl was very possessive of her brother, so I decided my only solution was to get my own Danny. I went home and begged my mother for a younger brother. She laughed it off, but I persisted, badgering her and my father for over a month for my very own Danny.

Lo and behold, my wish came true! Nine months later, my mother gave birth to a baby boy and my parents named him Danny. My excitement was endless! To this day, I remind him on every birthday that had it not been for me, he would not exist.

But there was a lesson my four-year-old mind picked up on—persistence pays off. I believed I could do anything I set my mind to. So, I focused on the energy and vibrancy of that furry-tailed squirrel.

Believe it or not, it worked! That image alone stuck in my subconscious, and while my hair did thin, it stayed mostly intact.

CHAPTER 13

Just Take Me Already

I went back to school in January 2006 while on the third round of the chemo cocktail. After one of the treatments, I was highly neutropenic (low white blood cell count), and that meant I should self-isolate due to the likelihood of becoming critically ill. I had missed so much school and needed to run by campus to pick up messages and assignments. It was going to be fifteen minutes at most I told myself. I wouldn't likely come in contact with many people, so I ignored my doctor and went to school to pick up my missed assignments without a face mask.

Little did I know there was a virus spreading through campus. I can only blame vanity for the reluctance to wear a mask. Cats are proud, and as they say, pride goeth before the fall. I was there for no more than twenty minutes. My doctor warned me that if I came down with a fever of 100.3°F or more, I would need to report immediately to the ER to get IV antibiotics and fluids. Failing to do this within six hours meant I would die of sepsis.

That midnight, I woke up with a 104°F temperature. I was sweating bullets. I popped some Tylenol and called the emergency number. The doctor on call said to come in immediately.

At this point, my health was at its worst. Every day was a deeper level of hell, and the only thing that kept me going was the stabbing pain in my heart at the image of my parents' faces if I left this world. Exhaustion sapped my energy every moment of every day. Cancer consumed my every thought. Will this treatment work? What will I do next? Will my heart give out before I can find my cure? I was in so much pain, I'd forgotten what it felt like *not* to be in pain.

I turned the phone off and lay back down. For twenty minutes, I just lay there, contemplating doing nothing. I wondered if this was the chance I needed to end the misery and let myself go in a quick and relatively peaceful manner. I was tired of being sick and didn't see an end to the suffering.

Just take me already, I prayed with anger fueled by exhaustion.

Then, God answered.

The anger turned into a burning in my stomach, a bitter revolt against the decision I was considering. The switch was sudden, as if injected into me from some outside force. I sat up in my bed and immediately knew what was happening. God was speaking to me, not so much in words but in a surety of life, in the *choice* to live.

There were no mistakes in life!

God was not done with me. There was a plan for this life, and I had to go through it all. All the suffering and hurt were there for a reason, to build my character, and more importantly, to build my trust in Him. In my lowest moments, God was nearest, holding me up.

I thought I had been at my worst. In that moment, I convinced myself that everything would look up, that I would make it through and survive this trial because God was there, guiding me. I still didn't know which path we were walking—take me or heal me—but I felt at peace with either one because on both journeys I was not alone.

I crawled out of bed, woke my parents, and asked them to drive me to the hospital.

As weak and ill as I was at that moment, I'd also never felt stronger. It's a good thing, too, because the kitten was about to need her claws.

Arriving at the hospital, I needed blood. I was tired and weak in a nuanced way only someone who has needed blood transfusions can understand. I instinctively knew my red blood cells were dangerously low, and I would crash soon. This was at about 6 a.m.

My doctor tested my blood and said my counts were normal.

"There's no way that can be accurate," I disagreed. "I'm weak, tired, shaky. I know my body. I've needed too many transfusions not to recognize the signs. Can you repeat the test?" I was out of breath, gasping for air. Even breathing was exhausting.

He never looked at my face, just kept scribbling on the chart and checking his phone. "Let's just keep an eye on you and see what happens." And with that, he disappeared.

As expected, I got worse. Mom was nudging me not to be rude to the doctor. I acquiesced. I held out a few more hours, but when my mom left, I had the doctor paged so I could reason with him.

He burst into my room after an hour, looking perturbed.

"I'm getting weaker," I persisted. I couldn't even sit up in bed to argue with him. "Will you at least repeat the blood test? Something is not right. I know it."

"Ma'am, there's no reason to doubt the blood work." It was like he was trying to convince a doubting ten-year-old there was a Santa Claus. "You have a high fever and that can leave you feeling drained. It explains the weakness. Continue fluids and Tylenol. That's all I can do for the moment." And again, he disappeared into the hallway with a flounce of his starched white coat.

I was so tired and weak I couldn't muster the energy to yell at him. I told myself to wait, and when the shift changed, I asked the next doctor to test my blood. He did, and found out I was dangerously anemic.

The previous doctor, so I was told, had my results confused with another patient's. To make things worse, my blood type is extremely rare, so by the time they finally placed the transfusion order, there was no blood left. I had to wait until more came in an emergency delivery from the Red Cross. I waited fourteen hours total for the transfusion.

This was only the beginning of what I would encounter during my stay, but it was part of the continuation of my transformation of Bisseh the Kitten to Bisseh the Tiger. Bisseh the Kitten sometimes needed to find support for a decision, or was too shy to ask for what she needed, but always knew she was capable of anything. However, Bisseh the Tiger had no issue demanding her needs be met.

When you're sick, you're at the mercy of an overworked, understaffed system. I had to learn to fight for myself, but some days I didn't like who I had to become to do that. Nor was I raised to be this way. I was not one to challenge. I was raised to respect others and respect authority. But when you're fighting for your life, all bets are off.

When I was admitted, I was told I would only be in for two to three days. I was there for nineteen days—almost three weeks of non-stop antibiotics and prepackaged foods. I was not allowed to eat anything unless it was completely sterile. Anyone entering my room had to wear a face mask.

Normal white blood cell counts are 1.0. My count was 0.03. My immune system was practically nonexistent. Ironically, I was fully functioning ... with pneumonia! I was coherent and walking around, and my doctor said he had never seen a patient with such a low blood count act so vibrant and awake.

One night, I was shivering while a fever of 103°F did a slow burn of my insides. I used the call button and told the nurse that I had a fever and was freezing cold. Rather than bringing me Tylenol, she simply turned the heat up in my room and walked out. I waited, thinking surely she would be back in a few minutes with my Tylenol. Ten minutes went by, then twenty, and finally, thirty minutes passed. I called her back.

"Are you going to bring me Tylenol?"

Her back stiffened and I could see her eyebrows knit together over the mask. "You never asked for Tylenol."

I'm ashamed to admit, but I lashed out at her. "I have septic blood and a 103 fever!" I said incredulously. "What exactly would you prescribe?"

She brought the Tylenol.

Then, there was the medical assistant with a bad case of smoker's cough. Every time she came into my room to take my temperature, she coughed in my face. The slightest infection could put me in a coma, and here she was, a hacking Joe Camel, like it wasn't a problem.

After one incident where I could smell the tuna she'd had for lunch, I waved her away. "Please don't cough in my face." I pointed to my chart and indicated the anti-infection protocol sign posted on the door. "Your cold would put me in the ICU."

"I'm not sick. I have allergies," she huffed, snatching up my chart.

"Do allergies keep you from covering your mouth when you cough, or is that simply bad manners?"

I know, not a moment I'm proud of, but my patience was as suppressed as my immune system by this time. Luckily, she was later caught in the act by a nurse and was transferred from my room.

On another occasion, I was awakened at 4 a.m. by a resident doing rounds so she could ask me if I was sexually active.

"How is that relevant at all to my situation?" I roared. "Get out and don't come back!"

She never did.

It was extremely difficult to rest in the hospital. What's the middle of the night to the patient is just the middle of a shift to a hospital worker. The nurses were always screaming, orderlies were laughing loudly, housekeeping was coming and going at all hours without any regard for the sick patients all around them.

I ended up leaving the hospital against medical advice (AMA), even though my cell count was still way below 1.0. How was I supposed to heal with no nutrition, no sleep, and the comedy of errors going on around me by all levels of staff? I was able to finish recovering at home—maybe it was the good night's rest I got every night and the nutritious food.

In March of that year, I went in for a routine scan, and the results showed I had a two-centimeter mass in the middle of my chest. It had not changed much from my previous scan, and the doctor wrote it off as inflammation. He did not follow up with a biopsy or PET scan. I'll never forget him saying, "Go home; you are healed."

I'll always remember the power of those words. Because I believed him. There was no way this crap show of a life could continue. There was no way it could happen *again*. Hope dangled within reach. Hope that the doctor knew what he was doing. My body was so broken there was no way cancer could survive. I really wanted to believe him, so I left and didn't look back. They'd nuked the heck out of me—I'd been gassed, radiated, burned, and toxified. What was left?

In reality, it was a dead mass with cancer cells hiding inside. They spread throughout my chest, into my lungs, and down my mediastinum . . . again. This was confirmed via a PET scan in June when my coughing and other symptoms returned. I now had cancer for the third time.

It was time to try something radically different.

Life #3

CHAPTER 14

Alternative Pathways

I doubled down on my research into alternative therapy programs, and this time, I would not be dissuaded by anything . . . or anybody. After all, I'd ignored my inner voice, a voice I half-believed was God nudging me in a certain direction, and all it had gotten me was another round of cancer spreading in my body like mold in a dark, damp basement.

It was time to find the light.

The irony of it all was that the treatments to cure my cancer had left my body a toxic mess, holistically unable to heal itself. Whatever I did next would not just need to heal my cancer, but first rebuild my body.

My family finally acknowledged that more chemotherapy was not the answer and maybe they should have listened to me. While it would be easy to scream, *I told you so!* at the top of my lungs, it did me no good. I also knew in my heart they'd done what they thought was best, and that was to fight the fight they knew from Loren's situation. They acted out of love. There was no room for blame, only healing. Healing the spirit went a long way toward healing the body as well.

I'd relied on my inner voice to lead me during my research for alternative treatments. I can't say I really knew what I was looking for in a clinic or a doctor. I wanted someone who would listen, who would treat *me* rather than my cancer.

I was looking into programs in Hawaii and realized they were too far and expensive when a program on *20/20* caught my eye. A nine-year-old boy had tried the traditional regimens to cure his cancer, but to no avail. The treatment was making him sicker. His parents were divorced, however, and while mom wanted to try alternative therapies, dad was suing to keep him in the traditional treatment programs. She was looking at child endangerment charges if she took her son out of the country to Mexico for treatment.

For me, however, it was if God were speaking to me personally. Finally, my prayers were answered.

I was an adult and could make my own choices; no one was going to subpoena me and drag me to court. But I had no real job by this point, and the salary from my summer job was spent on books and rent. While I was still a student, I relied on my parents to pay for any treatments. Luckily, they agreed that following the traditional path was not working.

The program reported on a healing center in Tijuana, Mexico, which coupled alternative treatments such as vitamins, minerals, and herbal supplements with special diets and lifestyle counseling, along with more conventional medical treatments when needed. They treated the entire patient, not just the cancer.

I immediately booked a flight to Mexico. My mother and I traveled together to meet with the doctors. Getting there was a little unnerving and, in retrospect, probably was not the safest. An unmarked white van picked us up at the airport. I'll admit, images from some bad action movies flashed through my head: the naïve Americans traveling to Tijuana, picked up by nefarious strangers and whisked away. Were we going to be kidnapped and held for ransom? We held each other's hands and prayed the entire way.

Thankfully, the drivers were legitimate, and we arrived at the hotel safely.

"Next time we'll take a cab," my mom whispered to me in a sigh of relief as we pulled into the hotel parking lot.

The next morning, we shuttled across the border and joined the dozens of new patients waiting to be examined. When I finally had my X-rays taken, I was told I was not the ideal candidate for the holistic brand of therapy alone. I had undergone too much chemo and radiation, and my immune system was too compromised.

The theory behind the elixir is that horses with cancer know instinctively which plants to eat. For centuries, herders watched and studied what the sick animals ate and turned this into the holistic remedies. I'd thought back to earlier instances where my body had craved cherries and seaweed, both natural remedies I needed at the time. As I read more and learned more about the treatment, I felt with certainty I was taking the right path, that I had followed God's voice inside my head and He had brought me here. All living beings are connected to our Creator.

Alternative, holistic treatments subscribe to a vastly different treatment method than traditional chemotherapy. Rather than a full-fledged *burn the entire forest to flush out the enemy* attack, they provide minerals, vitamins, and nutrients to strengthen and support the immune system so the body can fight the cancer itself, leaving all other naturally occurring cells alone. Since I'd undergone rigorous chemotherapy, my immune system was and forever will be compromised and unable to defend itself.

The doctor was clear that his prescribed tonic would probably not work as well as it would for a person who had not undergone chemotherapy and radiation. It's a double-edged sword. You listen to your doctors who tell you their treatments are necessary to save your life, only to find out those very treatments make you less able to thrive if you do survive the cancer. Despite the grim statistic, I walked away with a two-month supply of the tonic and supplements, with plans to renew the order until I was in remission.

I was desperate. I had left my New York doctors and their toxic regimens behind and believed this was the only option left to me. I believed God had led me to Mexico for a reason. I just had to discover the reason. My faith was hanging by a thread, but it was there.

So many things in my life up until now had pointed me to God wanting me to learn something from this experience. He had shown me I wasn't alone. The hairdresser's act of solidarity that day in the salon. The unwavering support of my family and friends who provided me with essentials like a home and food, necessities I barely had time to think about much less provide for myself.

But the cancer kept coming back.

If God was trying to tell me something, He was whispering. It's hard to hear a whisper in a raging storm.

My mom and I were feeling pretty low on the shuttle back to the hotel. In our silence, we overheard an older gentleman talking about how he had cancer and was being treated at another center, also in Tijuana, and really saw a benefit from his treatments. I knew this was the sign from God to have hope. My mother and I got the information and made an appointment for the next day.

We saw two doctors from the new center in their Tijuana office. One doctor was to monitor me day to day, and the other would see me once a week. He would monitor my viral loads and assess my immune system's reaction to the treatments. I was put on a strict diet called a Candida (yeast) Cleanse. In addition, I did daily blood ozone therapies and vitamin drips to kill fungus and viruses. I even peed into a cup, added powder to my urine to make it less acidic, and injected the pee back into my body. Yes, I was so desperate for a cure that I injected myself with my own urine!

Another radical treatment they prescribed—which, in retrospect, I should not have done—was to be injected with a dead virus. The theory was that this virus would stimulate my immune system, so my body would be strong enough to combat other foreign agents such as cancer. I was given this shot every two weeks and would go home and "wait out" the reaction. That reaction was fever. I was told not to use Tylenol or any fever reducer. I followed the instructions faithfully as if my life depended on it. On these nights, my temperature would reach up to 104 degrees.

I visited this clinic for treatments six days a week for eight weeks straight. My mom had to return to work, so she left to go back to New York after three days. It was hard for her to leave me, but I never resented her decision. She put all her trust in God and the doctors that I would be safe and on the road to healing. I was in California for a total of three months, the majority of that time spent shuttling across the Mexican border six days a week for treatments.

CHAPTER 15

A Priceless Find
at the Dollar Store

With my mother back in New York, I was squarely in the hands of God and the Mexican doctors in my adventure away from Western medicine. The latter had quickly diagnosed me with a thyroid condition, something the US doctors had not caught, though it had likely been caused by the MVP cocktail used during my second relapse. These same American doctors said the Mexican *quacks* would kill me.

Slowly but surely, during this process, I began to see God's hand more and more in my life.

First, I'd been led to Mexico, and while that wasn't a successful match, it led me to the second clinic. Now, I had faith God would surround me with the helping hands I needed, just as He had done when I was battling cancer the first time in New York. At least that was my hope. As I said, my faith was hanging on by a thread, but I was listening in the storm for any hint of God's voice. I wanted to hear His message, even if it was a whisper.

While at the hotel in San Diego, I frequently visted a nearby dollar store. I became friends with the Middle Eastern owner, Wael. My parents were skeptical about him at first and told me not to tell him about my health issues. They'd made strides in their thinking on traditional Western medicine and realizing it may not hold all the answers. Their views on keeping my illness a secret because of traditional Jordanian beliefs had not progressed as much.

However, I had moved on to a new phase in my independence where I followed my heart's guidance more. I'd learned to be more self-reliant when I'd gone off to college, then to law school. I knew I could trust my judgment, although the dutiful daughter in me respected the authority of my parents. Still, instinct pushed me to trust Wael.

In truth, I was desperate for any kind of friendship and connection.

My parents' desire to keep my illness a secret meant the vast majority of my family did not know the battle I was facing. The isolation had a detrimental effect on my mental health, and in some ways, I felt like my parents were putting their own fears ahead of my own needs, caring more about their reputation than they did about my own mental health. I know that's not true, by the way, but it's how it felt.

Truthfully, the situation sucked. My mom felt extreme guilt for having to leave me there alone with a hot pot, a supply of Ramen noodles, and no cable television. It was a no-win for anyone.

I told Wael why I was in San Diego and learned that he had a daughter with the same cancer I had! He was immediately sympathetic and very warm. We exchanged numbers, and he checked in on me frequently while I was in town. Because of his constant care, my parents warmed to him and he became a friend to the entire family. But even with my new friend, those first weeks in San Diego were lonely.

It was not really an environment conducive to making friends. I was on a mission to heal, not socialize. Healing takes all of your energy. I was again forced into a life of selfishness, but this time, my selfishness was hopefully going to reap better rewards. There was still the pressure to follow the rules, and between the diets and daily treatments, there were plenty. It was almost easier to do nothing than try and figure out what was allowed. I wanted to get better and go home in one piece. It was a lot for a twenty-five-year-old.

I was never good at sitting quietly; I am still not. I don't like sitting in the silence because of the emotions it makes me face, so I run away. Otherwise, I would be plagued with thoughts of *How did I get here? What wrong turn did I take to land me in this hell?*

Each morning, I would take the clinic shuttle to Mexico alone, spend three hours a day there with little interaction, then shuttle back to my empty hotel. I ate dinner alone at the end of each isolated day, then went to sleep, having spoken only to doctors and their staff. Loneliness wears on a person, much like illness. I did what I could to keep my spirits up— talked to my family, studied, watched movies. This was before Netflix and Hulu were available, and six channels of basic cable didn't lend to entertainment or escape.

It's easy to feel abandoned at times like that. There's something to be said for connecting with people when you're facing such a hard disease.

Especially people fighting the same fight you face daily.

I thought back to another time when the loneliness had weighed on me so heavily. In fact, it weighed so heavily it had taken me to the floor in a fancy French restaurant on New Year's Eve. So, I returned to the prayer I'd whimpered that day.

Help me understand.

I had to believe God was silencing the noise around me so I could hear His whispers. I just needed to listen closely. So, I waited for a sign.

Then I heard about a living arrangement from a doctor at the clinic. A man owned a large house on the beach and rented out rooms to patients from the clinic. You can't imagine my excitement! I called him up as soon as I learned about the place, and to my delight, there was a room available. I secured it instantly and moved out of the hotel and into the house the very next day. It was perfect! An early version of Airbnb. I shared the home with other patients going to the same clinic. Our free transport took us there together in the morning and returned us home in the evenings. The price of our rent provided food, but it also included a private chef. Although we were all battling different illnesses, we had community. I spent the evenings and weekends walking on the beach, enjoying the serenity.

Another prayer was answered. I think that was the message I needed to learn from this experience. I wasn't alone, even when it felt like I was. And that God would provide for my needs. I needed to learn to remember that, to have faith in God's presence in my life.

After three months in California, I returned home looking like a typical cancer patient—gaunt, pale, and lethargic. My weight had dropped to 118 pounds, a fifteen-pound drop that was very noticeable on my 5'7" frame, due to the strict diet.

The theory was that cancer likes sugar, so I had to remove sugar from my diet to starve it . . . no more simple carbohydrates, including fruit, bread, pasta, and rice. I lived on high protein and vegetables. I also could not have anything with yeast or acid. For the tincture to work, I had to keep my body neutral, so as not to dilute its effectiveness. I could not eat anything acidic, which included tomatoes, lemons, and vinegar.

At times, it seemed like medicine was the biggest part of my diet. I had to bring about a dozen bags of pills and potions back to New York. I also brought my diet back with me and wasn't tempted to cheat. As long as I kept to the regimen, the cancer would remain in check. I had stopped all chemo and other treatments synonymous with Western medicine, and this was my last and only hope to survive.

One afternoon, I went to grab brunch with my friends. I'm sure as they listened to my cobbled together food order, it must have sounded something like a scene out of *When Harry Met Sally*. My friends didn't seem to mind, but I found it an exhausting ritual. My life was funny in a sad kind of way, or maybe it was sad in a funny kind of way. I'm not really sure which.

I did believe this new program was putting me on the path back to health, but everything comes at a price.

During my stay in Mexico, I had missed my cousin's wedding. She didn't even know I had cancer; three years into this nightmare and we were still actively hiding it from the extended family. She thought I was at some study abroad program. I missed the first six weeks of law school, *and* I had picked up a virus toward the end of my stay in Mexico because of my weak immune system. It hung around for two weeks after I returned to New York, so I had to miss my best friend's wedding in North Carolina as well.

It felt like I couldn't catch a break! Isn't one sickness enough? *Why me?* I silently shouted to the heavens. *Why not me?* the heavens seemed to shout back. I wasn't even a full-fledged lawyer yet, but I was already losing arguments for lack of evidentiary support.

But as I stuck to the regimen, things started to get better. I was eating healthy, feeling stronger, and school was going great. Only one semester behind, I was able to catch up in my studies and graduate from law school in December 2006. At the start of the new year, I was offered a job to work with my older brother's mortgage company.

In the last week of January 2007, I moved into an apartment in Manhattan. I was hanging out with my friends and enjoying being free and making money. I was still going for scans every three months, as was protocol for the past two years, but they consistently showed that the mass was slowly shrinking. Life was finally looking up.

It's almost like I should have known better.

Because once again, like clockwork, my world fell apart.

Life #4

CHAPTER 16:

Shaken, Not Stirred

In February 2007, I went in for my routine scan. Dr. W came to my exam room looking neutral, which must be a class they teach in medical school: how to deliver bad news with a poker face.

"The cancer has spread, Rinad." He held my chart like a hand of cards he didn't want the opposing player to see, as if it would reveal something he was afraid to share. "At your last PET, you had a few spots in your lungs and stomach. Now it's moved into several areas of the chest, the right lung, and down through the abdominal cavity, even into the spleen and bones." The poker face faded a touch as the final card revealed a busted flush. "I'm sorry, but it's officially in Stage 4."

I'm sure he said something after that—something about treatment or plans or getting my affairs in order—all that *next step stuff* doctors are good at saying, but quite frankly, I didn't hear a word of it. I left the office with a high-pitched wail in my ears.

Help me understand.

I stumbled from the office, those words ringing in my ears: *officially in Stage 4.*

Help me understand.

I'd listened. I'd followed my heart. I'd gone to Mexico. I'd stopped shooting toxic chemicals into my body, letting it heal, letting nature deal with the cancer.

Help me understand.

My faith was shaken, but not broken. If I'd learned anything, I'd learned that faith can be a process just as understanding can be a process. Too often, people think of faith as an on-off switch. Faith is a cup to be filled over a lifetime. Sometimes it spills.

At the same time, I began experiencing severe sharp pains in my right chest, accompanied by shortness of breath. An X-ray showed that my lung was 30 percent effaced—one of the tumors was eating away at the lining of my right lung, causing a partial collapse. After examining me, my primary care physician (PCP) advised that if my shortness of breath got worse, I should go to the emergency room.

He didn't, however, mention anything about plane rides.

I told myself that if the shortness of breath got worse, I would follow my PCP's advice and go to the emergency room. But since at that moment I was breathing fine, I decided to hop on a plane to visit a friend in Miami . . . and nearly died three times in the process.

As soon as the plane took off, I felt like I was being choked and began to cough. It lasted the entire flight. I was in and out of the bathroom the whole time, trying to catch my breath. During one episode, I was in there so long the flight attendant used her key to open the door. She said she had been banging on the door, but I could not hear it over the coughing. Once in Miami, the cough never stopped, and I experienced the same coughing fits on both plane rides back to New York.

Arriving home, I spoke to my attending oncologist.

"I'd like to find a holistic treatment program in Mexico for my lungs. Are there any you would recommend?"

He looked doubtful. "Even if you could find one you liked, you'll be unable to fly with a pneumothorax. The pressurized cabin in the plane would cause serious issues with a collapsed lung."

"I just returned from Miami," I explained and he nearly choked on his surprise.

"I'm going to refer you to a cardiothoracic surgeon for more information about addressing the lung issues, but for now, stay off of airplanes."

That surgeon still discusses me at conferences, calling me a "medical marvel" for surviving three plane rides with a severely collapsed lung.

I confronted my PCP about his not informing me to avoid planes and not sending me to the ER after the scan results.

"I didn't ask you to go to the ER because I knew you wouldn't," he said. He obviously had been speaking to Dr. W about my refusal of chemo and other traditional treatments. "And frankly, I didn't warn you about plane rides because I didn't think anyone in *your condition* would even think to go on vacation."

I dropped him from being my doctor immediately. I had once

again survived my run-in with traditional medicine, and again, survived another test with people. I've admitted before to having strong opinions, and I make no apologies for my perfectionist tendencies. I know that can make me a difficult person to deal with sometimes. However, I'd like to think a doctor would also tend toward perfectionism. Guessing how a patient will react to news or presuming what a patient will or will not do in a given set of circumstances in a medical crisis seems arrogant at its best, and dangerous at its worst.

That weekend, I admitted myself to the hospital to have my lung inflated. A small tube was inserted into my lung, sewn into place, and attached to a machine that pumped air into the lung to inflate it over time. I was attached to it for three days straight.

After the bombshell news from Dr. W about my cancer moving to Stage 4, dating once again replaced the part of my life taken over by chemo and life-and-death decisions. It allowed me to be Rinad the Law Student or Rinad the Twenty-Something New Yorker rather than Rinad the Cancer Patient. It also supplemented a part of my life hidden by my family's continued reluctance to be open and honest about my cancer diagnosis. It was temporarily filling the gaping hole that the big C kept ripping open.

I'd talked about the isolation caused by the secrecy of my illness within the family. Dating filled that void, at least in part. I was meeting people and making social connections, even if I wasn't telling them about my cancer. It was my escape.

That was the year I met Harold. He lived in the W Hotel in Times Square because he did a lot of bicoastal traveling and living out of hotels was easier for him to conduct business. He was a sports agent and baseball scout, and regularly traveled to Los Angeles, New York, and the Dominican Republic. He was stylish and cute.

We met at the W Hotel bar. I was attracted to his bright smile and fancy suit. It turned out that's all he ever wore: suits with a smile. He owned five of them, and that was it, so I never saw him in anything else.

The weekend I stayed at the hospital getting my lung reinflated, I told Harold I had gone to DC to visit friends. I wasn't ready to tell him about my condition. I quickly learned from my experience with Jake that telling the truth doesn't end well, so I continued with the deception. It came natural to me because I was doing the same thing with my family and friends. I got so used to lying to everyone about my health that I didn't even feel guilty. I was released on a Monday afternoon, went home, showered, and met him for dinner that evening.

Right before I got the clearance to be discharged, Dr W visited me to discuss next steps regarding my lymphoma.

"You know the situation, Rinad," he said, looking as serious as I'd ever seen him. "I believe the only thing that can save you now is a bone marrow transplant. I think you should begin the testing for marrow immediately."

I shook my head. "I'm going back to Mexico after my discharge. I want to give the holistic treatment at the center another try."

Dr. W closed my chart and tucked it under his arm. "I think those treatments are why you're sitting here now, your cancer spreading as it is, so I'm against the alternative therapies you're proposing." Then very sternly, he added, "If you do not follow the regimen I've prescribed, I can't continue to be your doctor. It's my opinion that you won't live more than three months as things are now." I could tell it was hurting him to say this as much as it was for me to hear it. Then he turned and walked out of the room.

CHAPTER 17

Too Good to Be True

A month later, my lung collapsed again, this time worse than before. The tumor had grown and eaten away at the pleural lining—that's what attaches the lung to the diaphragm. I was set to return to Mexico, but needed another surgery to survive the plane ride.

The procedure, a cementation, was more invasive than the previous. Because of that, I insisted it be performed by the actual cardiothoracic surgeon, but was refused. Since I was in a teaching hospital, a resident had to perform the procedure. I wanted to leave, but at that point, I was already cut open with a tube sticking out of my body, so I acquiesced. I had zero bargaining power.

I stayed attached to the machine pumping air through a tube into my lung for three days straight, but the lung could no longer support itself. The doctors had to cement the lung itself to the lung cavity. Imagine feeling your lung glued to your ribs. They literally poured cement, called talc, through a tube into my body to glue me together.

When I came out of anesthesia, the pain was excruciating, like nothing I'd ever experienced. Imagine seeing color for the first time, only that color was pain. I screamed and writhed, gasping for each breath. Every breath I took felt like someone was trying to rip me in half from the inside.

This pain only made me realize how lonely and alone I was feeling. As a Christian, I believed we should be in community with one another. We were not meant to do life alone. We see that in our earliest lessons; God put us on this earth as two, Adam and Eve. I wanted a husband by my side more than ever in that moment.

Since I was still single, I needed my parents' help. But I wanted to be an adult, to live free and make my own decisions. I was back to the Catch-22 of my life. They couldn't leave their jobs to jump to my side every time I had an appointment; they'd already been doing that for many years. At the same time, I was their daughter. Where do you draw the line between child and adult?

I woke up from surgery to a roommate I'd never met before. After listening to my wails of pain, even she called the nurse to bring me pain medication.

An hour and a half later, it arrived.

I later learned that the resident made two critical errors. First, she should have known I would be in a great deal of pain coming out of the procedure and should have had pain medication ready immediately. Second, the nurse assisting said the tube had moved during the procedure, allowing the talc to spill inside of me. This was causing the majority of the immense pain.

But I guess she wasn't supposed to tell me that because, in an effort to diffuse the situation, the surgeon contradicted the nurse's story saying that the procedure *was* performed correctly and that in 5 percent of cases, patients have a severe reaction to the talc. *To this day*, I have cement lodged in my lung and have difficulty breathing due to the permanent scars it created.

Because I was in the hospital for a longer period, I lied to Harold again, telling him I had bronchitis, and the cough was so bad that it had collapsed my lung. He bought it, as usual. Part of me questioned his commitment to me and our relationship if he could so easily buy my lies. But a bigger part of me questioned my own humanity at lying to someone I supposedly cared about. I kept coming back to believing it was a personal decision. I wasn't ready to share this part of myself with him, but I was still holding back the most vital part of myself. How could I expect to find a real commitment if I wasn't being completely honest about who I was?

In reality, though, it was fear. Fear that he would disappear like others had done in the past. Fear that he would look at me differently. I didn't want the two parts of my life, my two identities, to blur. Harold was in the *other* part of my life, the part not tainted by the cancer diagnosis. In that life, there were no chemo treatments or bone marrow transplants or clocks ticking down my time left on earth. I wasn't ready to give that up.

For months, every time I took a breath, I felt sharp stabbing pains in my side, the same kind felt by people with multiple broken ribs. But

I had a bigger problem—the cementation hadn't worked. My lung was still collapsing. It happened two more times, making the total count four. Once, it happened while I was at a Cinco de Mayo party. All I had done was laugh.

I was again at a crossroads as to how to treat the cancer. The pain after surgery was insurmountable. The lung was not inflating on its own, so the trip to Mexico was not feasible. For the first time, doing nothing was a viable option. It may have been my most viable option, but that's not what I did.

My brother was engaged to be married that summer in Turkey and my sister in the fall, well beyond the three months Dr. W. had given me in March if I abstained from his regimen of chemo. Had I not had familial responsibilities, I might have opted to terminate all treatments and live out the rest of my days traveling and enjoying life with my friends and family. But I couldn't, knowing my illness and possible death would be a specter on their day of happiness.

At least that is what I was telling myself. Being completely honest, even with all the doom and gloom on the horizon, there was a stronger force pushing me forward. I had hope. Hope I would find a cure. Hope I would find my forever person. This was the real reason I was still fighting. I still had that dream of getting married one day. That desire fueled every decision.

Turkey seemed unlikely, but I wanted to try. After the lung collapse in May, it was questionable whether I could even make it to the July wedding. I was absolutely not going through the talc surgery again and did not want to risk getting on a plane—one can push their luck only so many times. The tiger dug in her claws. I was going to make these weddings.

So, we watched, and we waited, and we prayed.

It often sounds like prayer is a final option for me. It's not. Prayer became a continual mantra in my head throughout the day. *Help me understand. Help me find strength. Help me see the path You have chosen for me.* I had long ago given up the belief that I was in charge. I knew, without any doubt, that God was calling the shots. My job was to silence the noise of fear and doubt and distrust and let Him show me what I needed to see. *What am I not seeing? Not understanding?*

The whispering voice became louder and easier to hear at times.

Faith is like standing at the back of a theater listening to a full orchestra. Sometimes, the orchestra is playing a classical piece and the ebb and flow of the instruments makes it easy to pick out the woodwinds from the brass and the timpani is a solid but supporting force in the background. Other times, you're listening to the frenzied clash of notes because the woodwinds are playing heavy metal freakbeat and the brass is playing avant-garde punk death-grind while percussion whips up a thrashcore rhythm on a different beat.

Regardless of what the orchestra played, I listened. I didn't always understand the song, but I knew it was music. That was faith to me. I didn't always know what God was telling me, but I trusted there was a message.

Luckily, dare I say miraculously, the lung inflated on its own. I was able to travel to Turkey to see my brother get married, although I didn't push my luck and waited until the last minute to book my ticket. I shared the day with my family and celebrated this new beginning for my brother. I knew there would be grandchildren to carry on the family name, the traditions we'd brought with us from Jordan, the new traditions we'd learned in America. I knew my parents would have somewhere to focus their love and energy in the future.

I was also thinking of my own future. I was now well beyond Dr. W's estimated ninety-day timeline handed down in March. I was living on borrowed time.

There's a thin line between hope and despair when you are facing an illness such as cancer. When you hear a doctor give you three months to live, you can start counting the hours, or you can just live each day without worrying about what comes next. In truth, cancer or not, you never really know how many tomorrows are in your calendar.

When I returned to New York, I spoke to Wael, my friend in San Ysidro, who put me in touch with a woman named Joyce. Joyce was an agent who matched Americans up with Mexican doctors offering alternative therapies. That's how I met Dr. V, who said he could cure me—completely *cure* me—after two weeks of treatments.

He'd seen my scans and recommended I do a combined chemo and radiation regimen, but do half the dosage traditionally administered in the United States so I would not suffer the violent nausea and hair loss. The main difference was he would add holistic therapies to allow the chemo to work better.

My sister's warning from my last foray into alternative treatments played in my head. *Time is crucial, Rinad. You cannot take any chances with feel-good, New Age wannabe doctors who just want to take you for every penny.*

I was already out of time and money. I didn't think I had much more to lose.

I was on a plane back to Mexico two days later and began treatment the day I touched down.

For two weeks, I had radiation treatments from my chest down to my stomach. Dr. V used half the chemo dosage as normally prescribed and put laetrile (an enzyme found in apricot pits) in the cocktail with other natural pills, which counteracted the nausea so I didn't experience the vomiting normally associated with chemo. I never lost my appetite and was able to eat full meals every day. I also didn't need the Procrit shots or blood transfusions.

My father accompanied me this time. We stayed with Wael and his family, and he drove us over the border every day. He made me promise not to tell his daughter, who shared my diagnosis, that this was my third relapse. He didn't want to scare her. This is something I would encounter again later, after my return to New York when searching for a support group, and it's something I would struggle with accepting. My story scares people.

Remember that thin line between hope and despair I mentioned earlier? For me, it was like looking at Loren as a mirror to my own diagnosis. I expected my disease to run the same course as hers and, as we all know, that couldn't be further from the truth. I think Wael was worried his daughter would look at me, fighting my third relapse and barely hanging on, and see a potential path for her own cancer. It sounded terrifying even to me.

He wanted her to hold on to the hope side of the line as long as possible.

So, I told her it was my first bout with cancer. I was already lying to everyone else about my health; what was one more? And it was the least I could do to thank Wael for his generosity and kindness. It was challenging at times talking with his daughter. She did not think it fair she had to go through the full chemo regimen—the same kind I did the first time around—and that I get to be treated for only two weeks, and never lose my hair, or become extremely sick, and would still be cured.

How I bit my tongue!

But like her father, I wanted to protect her from the truth.

It was also the moment I realized my parents were trying to protect me by keeping the cancer a secret. The fiercest instinct for a parent is to protect their child. By guarding the status of my health, they protected me from well-meaning but sometimes ignorant comments, intrusive questions, or insensitive remarks. Just like Wael's daughter didn't understand the difference in our treatment plans and saw unfairness, I had the benefit of seeing the whole picture. Looking back, I see now how my parents were keeping me guarded in their love because they had the whole picture before them.

As I prepared to leave the Mexican clinic, Dr. V informed me he needed to extend the original prescribed treatment, citing that my body had been severely compromised by previous treatments. Two weeks was not going to be enough to put me in remission. Nor was the original dosage going to be sufficient for his promised cure.

It was difficult learning the promises made by Dr. V were hollow. It's easy in hindsight to say, *Anything that sounds too good to be true probably is,* but that would be too simplistic a judgment. I was not hoping for a good deal on a used car. I was fighting for my life, and not for the first time. I'd not jumped straight to outlandish promises from a foreign doctor immediately after hearing my diagnosis back in 2003. I'd followed the traditional treatment plans. I'd pumped toxins into my body and used radiation to kill the cancer cells, along with a good portion of healthy cells.

Nothing had worked.

So, when a doctor dangled the word *cure,* I jumped on a plane. I've always been a reasonably intelligent person. Desperation shoved common sense and rationale right out the window. My hope for a cure outweighed any red flags I might have felt about Dr. V's treatment plan.

Remember, these were not days I'd thought I'd be around to see. Dr. W was one of the doctors I'd trusted, so when he gave me three months, I believed him. Each day I was sick crossed one more day off the very small calendar of days I'd been given by the doctor. All of those days had a big red X.

I also wanted to believe this could be an answer to my prayer. I still thought of faith in terms of rewards. *Follow the rules. Get my prize.* My desperation went beyond the physical. It dug into the spiritual. I needed to see a physical manifestation that my faith was not in vain.

Sitting in Dr. V's office that last day was like sitting on the edge of a cliff with the ground crumbling beneath my butt.

"You'll need another two rounds of my prescribed regimen. These will be delivered six weeks apart." Like most doctors, Dr. V delivered the news as if he expected me to simply follow directions, like a faithful dog following the master's command. He didn't even bother to look up from the notes he was making in my file. He was the doctor, after all. Who was I? No one. I was simply the person who was dying.

"No."

It's funny how such a small word can elicit such a big reaction. He paused the scribbling, lifting his head as if I'd done a surprising trick. "What do you mean?"

"I'm not going to spend another twelve weeks here. My flight back to the US leaves in the morning. You knew my condition before I arrived and promised me a cure based on that information. Now you want to extend the treatment?"

There's a look doctors use—a slight tilt of the head, a half-smile, a narrowing of the eyes—when they're patronizing a patient but don't want to seem patronizing. That was the look I received from Dr. V. "The body doesn't always respond as we hope, Rinad."

Anger leaked into my voice. "Then you should have said that when you promised me a cure."

In truth, the anger was equally shared between us. No, he should not have promised me something he could not deliver. And I should not have believed his promise. The red flags were there, but I chose not to see them or heed the inner voice that warned me about following this course of treatment.

Desperation, thy name is Rinad.

In the end, we reached a compromise. He gave me a prescription for the additional treatments and I promised to find a doctor to carry them out. I was dying. I had nothing left to lose at this point.

Luckily, a friend of my brother was an oncologist and agreed to give me the prescribed medicine when I returned to New York. In addition to a longer dosage, I learned Dr. V put me on a higher dose of chemo without my knowledge. My Spanish was a little rusty.

I became suspicious when I returned home and my hair started falling out in clumps. When I called him, he explained the natural agents had not been working effectively because of the damage done by my previous treatments . . . so he had upped the chemo dosage. Apparently, he didn't feel the need to inform me of the change in treatment.

I was appalled. What I learned, however, was that he was under no obligation to inform me, the patient, of his decision. In the United States, doctors are not allowed to change the agreed-upon treatment without informed consent from the patient. In Mexico, there are few rules. Their protocols for patient notification are more like guidelines rather than requirements.

I also later learned that in Mexico, Dr. V increased the radiation dosage without consent, which would eventually cause my heart failure.

Every part of his treatment regimen was compromised and distorted. Over time, my perfect ejection fraction—the measure of how much of the heart's blood capacity leaves the heart with each pump—fell from 60 to 20 percent, which necessitated a heart transplant.

During all the shuttling back and forth over the Mexican border, I was still dating Harold. I told him I was in California at a training conference for work. He was traveling between New York and the Dominican Republic, so it wasn't difficult to maintain the illusion.

I felt guilty talking to him every night as I walked back across the border to San Ysidro. I would tell him about the fictitious people I met and the different activities we did in fake training. Even so, I looked forward to talking to him every night. That fictional world was my only break from the disaster that had become my reality. I really relied on him.

But eventually, I came clean with him. He was shocked that I had kept such a huge secret from him, but not upset, and understood my need for privacy. I think I might have been more shocked by his understanding than he was of my lies.

It was really my first positive experience since Ajay in terms of dating and the truth of my cancer. I knew there were people who would not run from my side when I told them I had cancer, but they mostly fell safely into the friend category. Romantic interest was a different ballgame. Ajay had been the ideal in terms of support during my illness.

Jake, on the other hand, had run for the hills and never looked back. Harold wasn't running, at least not yet. I was now two for one in terms of dates-who-knew-and-stayed and dates-who-knew-and-ran. It wasn't much of a scientific sampling, but it's something that sticks with you.

To my dismay, after returning a second time from Mexico, new symptoms emerged. Walking down the street, I began gasping for air like someone was smothering me. I assumed my lung had collapsed again, but to my horror, the reality was far worse.

Due to the cumulative damage of all my past treatments, I had gone into a state of respiratory distress. Large areas of my lung had become hardened, no longer allowing air to pass freely through. Over the next few months, I was unable to climb stairs, and there were periods of time when I couldn't even walk. I would be bedridden for days at a time, and my life became tethered to an oxygen tank.

The only good thing about being bedridden was that I spent time reading the Bible, looking for guidance and sustenance for my wavering faith. I wanted peace. I wanted answers. I wanted what I would not find in the words written there: God's reasoning behind letting all of this happen. But it doesn't work that way, does it? Scraping together the very last vestiges of strength I could muster, I kept pushing forward, trusting the right path would be revealed.

My oncologist referred me to a pulmonologist named Dr. M. She took my history, did a physical, and without ordering any tests, diagnosed me with pulmonary fibrosis, secondary to Bleomycin (the "B" in ABVD) toxicity. She said there was nothing that could be done and I would always have trouble breathing. Again, without any tests, she also told me I had asthma and gave me an inhaler. I used the inhaler for months without relief.

I went to see my brother's friend, the oncologist, for the last two rounds of chemotherapy Dr. V had prescribed. When he saw the prescription, he said it would not be enough to put me in remission, I needed a far more aggressive treatment, and my only hope was a bone marrow transplant. What irony! The only procedure that could save my life was a bone marrow transplant, but my heart and lungs were too weak to endure the procedure; it would most likely kill me.

As an alternative—not really any alternative, but my only other option—the doctor said I could do the chemo as maintenance, every couple of months, for the rest of my life. The reality of that route sunk in, of me being in and out of hospitals, enduring more blood transfusions, having constant nausea, and being perpetually bald. I passed. I was done with simply "prolonging life."

CHAPTER 18

The Shack

After more soul-searching, I still had not found peace in my situation. You might think I would have become numb, but the opposite was true. Every diagnosis was a new whirlwind of trauma, causing me to question each decision I'd made before it. I would feel rage, regret, and disappointment—sometimes all at once—over the lack of success with the treatments. There is an absence of humanity in the treatments hurled at patients from doctors who likely couldn't remember the patient's name without a chart in front of them.

Adding to the cacophony of emotional turmoil, I was in intense pain. I became isolated, not wanting to inflict my sour disposition on others. Through it all, I had only a few true friends. People would come around while I was healthy . . . and steer clear while I was sick.

I think for many people, the inability to help in a situation like mine brings guilt to the surface. Trust me, if you know someone fighting a life-or-death illness, they're not expecting miracles from you. We also want to sit and talk about something other than the disease wreaking havoc on our lives.

Among my few supportive friends was Jeanne, whom I had stayed in touch with since graduating from law school. She has been a great support while I've traveled this winding and twisty road toward a cure for my cancer. She has always validated my feelings and shared my distrust of the health care industry.

During the summer of 2007, Jeanne and I were going to meet up for a picnic in scenic Long Island. The train schedules were messed up that day, so I ended up missing my train by thirty seconds and had to wait another hour and forty-five minutes for the next one. Although I was disappointed, it turned out to be a blessing in disguise.

I decided to wait out my misfortune in a bookstore and came across a book called *The Shack*. It was about answering the first question that pops into our head when tragedy strikes: Why me?

Sound familiar?

It dealt with why God lets bad things happen to good people. I paused over the book's cover. It claimed to answer that exact question I'd been mulling over in my mind for years. For a moment, I debated. Did I really want to know the answer? God's reason may not be something I would like. God, however, had guided me into that bookstore, to that very book. I purchased it.

It was a tragic story of a man whose five-year-old daughter was savagely murdered. Overtaken by grief, he received a letter in the mail addressed from God, asking him to meet in the same cabin where his daughter's blood-soaked dress had been found. Hoping it was actually a letter from the killer taunting him, the man headed out to the cabin to get revenge.

Instead of finding the killer, he met Jesus, God, and the Holy Spirit in the cabin. He spent a weekend with Them, asking how They could allow such an awful thing to happen when They claimed to love him so much.

Even after so many years of Bible study and attending church, I really hadn't understood God's love. I had never really felt it, and it took me years to accept the notion that God can love you and still allow bad things to happen. In reality, God's love and blessings aren't void of pain and suffering. They aren't mutually exclusive. I read that book half-a-dozen times to fully understand why He permits these things. It is *because* He loves us, because we are closest to Him when we are furthest from comfort.

And to be close to God brings real comfort.

I'd seen this truth in my life several times, from that New Year's Eve huddled in the bathroom of the French restaurant to the loneliness and fear and isolation during my time in Mexico when I had no one to lean on but myself and my faith.

There's a poem I've read called "Footprints" about a man walking along the beach. He sees two sets of footprints in the sand, one belonging to him and another belonging to God. Then, at the lowest points of his life, he sees only one set of footprints. He calls out and asks how God could abandon him. God says when he only sees one set of footprints, the man was not walking alone. That was when God was carrying him.

The Shack was a similar story about God's amazing love for His children and how He carried them through the difficult times. He even loved those who made horrible, evil decisions that affected others, leaving them free to make their own choices. He loves us even in our mistakes.

Reading this book helped me realize that everything was bigger than me. If God was calling me to Heaven, I was not going to accomplish anything by fighting the cancer. I would only be delaying the inevitable and making myself miserable in the process. I believed God had a plan for me so I should leave my fate with Him. That's where I would be safest. As soon as He decided it was time for me to go, then it would be my time, and not because I chose one treatment over another. That is why I was so uneasy with every decision I ever made. Doubting and second-guessing; I was focusing on the wrong cure.

After lunch, while sitting on the hammock in Jeanne's yard, I told her my decision.

"I'm done with treatments, Jeanne." I watched her reaction from the corner of my eye, not sure if she would accept the news or, like my family, fight me on it.

She sighed, leaning her shoulder against mine. "Oh, dear one. I can't say I like it, but I know how much you've been through the last few years. If this is your decision, then I'm behind you 1,000 percent. Whatever you need, count me in."

I felt like a great weight had been lifted knowing I had someone in my corner, and I felt better than I had for months. Looking back now, I do not have a single regret about stopping treatments. I never worried about dying. I didn't want to die, but I'd seen that God would be waiting to lift me from the pain. As Christians, our faith gives us the strength to endure, knowing we are not alone on the journey.

On the contrary, the earlier decisions I had made, the recommendations of all the doctors, caused my anxiety. I'd been left alone time and time again to make almost impossible life-and-death decisions about the course of my treatment. It was the classic no-win situation.

Once I left behind those recommendations, for the first time I felt that true *"peace that surpasses all understanding."* (Philippians 4:7)

I completed the two rounds of treatments the Mexican doctor had prescribed, then told my oncologist no more. And he informed me in no uncertain terms that if I refused to continue, I would only have six months to a year to live. I smiled, thanked him for his time, and walked out of his office, never to return again.

CHAPTER 19

Facing the Music

I waited until after my brother's wedding in July to tell my family I had decided to stop treatments. I was scared of their reaction and sad that my brother's wedding might be the last vacation we would take together as a family. On the whole, though, for the first time in years, I was truly happy. Not the fake kind of happiness you paint on like makeup when you want to forget your problems, but an overwhelming, overflowing peace and contentment.

Here I was at twenty-seven, facing the almost certainty of an early, untimely end of my life, and I'd found peace with the decision. It was one of the most bittersweet moments of my life.

I called Pastor Tom, my family pastor and health care proxy, and asked him to come with me to tell my parents. My parents had been a large part of my continuation of the treatments, but now that I was making decisions based on my own reasoning, I needed to know my wishes would be carried out. With Tom acting as my health care proxy, I had the assurance my wishes would come first.

But telling my parents would not be easy. In the same way I had initially accepted their efforts to find me a husband in the traditional Jordanian way, I had accepted their guidance on the course of treatment to follow with my cancer. They'd made these decisions before when Loren was diagnosed and had met with success. It made sense to let that knowledge play a role in my decision-making.

I was not Loren, however, and I was not finding success in the traditional course of treatments. My physical health was deteriorating, but my mental health had never been stronger because I'd stood up for myself with the doctors. I'd rediscovered who I was at my core.

It was time, once again, to put my foot down.

On the night we'd planned to tell my parents, Pastor Tom came to the door, unannounced. Always the polite hosts, my parents let him in and offered refreshments. We all sat awkwardly on the couch at first, not speaking. My parents did not want to seem rude and ask why he was there, so I choked up an explanation.

"I asked Pastor Tom over to discuss something that's been on my heart. I hope you can listen with an open mind."

They looked at each other, then at us, but remained silent.

I told them. The words spilled out of me like a cup had overturned. I told them of the decision to stop treatments, that I thought God had brought me this far for a reason and now I just had to wait to see how the journey ended. I would either get better, stay the same, or I wouldn't.

My heart was in my throat and I could barely breathe, and for the first time not because of my lungs compromised by cancer and all the treatments! Would they fight me? Cry? Scream?

Pastor Tom leaned forward, his arms braced on his knees. "Rinad has prayed long and hard about this, and I have faith in her belief that God is guiding her in this journey."

To my surprise, they were calm. "And we have faith in her," my mother said, coming to sit by my side.

My father nodded, though I could see him fighting the tears as he cleared his throat. "If you have been praying about this, and if this was what you believe God wants from you, then we support your decision."

I couldn't believe it! They were not hysterical, upset, or emotional at all. Later that week, I told my sister . . . and that did not go as well.

"You're giving up! You want to die." She threw her hands up and paced the confines of the living room like a caged animal. "This is not the Bisseh we have raised you to be. This is a mistake! Baba did not raise us to make mistakes!" Her voice filled the house like his had on so many occasions.

I was sitting on the sofa next to her husband, watching her pace and fidget. I'd expected her to be upset and wanted her to understand my choices. "I have been fighting for four years, Loren. I did not make this decision on a whim." I went to her, putting my body in her path so she would face me and hopefully see the peace in my heart reflected on my face. "It is something I have thought and prayed about for a very long time."

"Then you are not listening to God's words correctly because I cannot believe He wants you to end your life like this."

We continued to argue as only sisters can. She was older and was used to me taking her advice without question. When other people were hanging out with their friends, we'd had only each other. No matter how I explained my perspective and reasons, she couldn't come to terms with it.

I don't blame her. She was stressed and had a lot on her plate. She was also trying to protect me, to be there by my side.

If I had been in her shoes, I'm certain my reaction would have been a lot worse. At the time I gave her the news, she was planning her fall wedding. I would learn years later Loren's wedding was originally scheduled for the following the year, but when I'd received the Stage 4 prognosis, she'd moved up the date so I would be able to serve as her maid of honor.

With the decision to ride out the rest of my days without cancer treatment, my PCP advised I see various specialists with the goal of improving the quality of my remaining life. In August 2008, I went to a palliative care center, which treats "end of life" patients. They prescribed a weekly massage. Amazingly, of all the massage specialists I could have been assigned to, I was assigned to *the one* who lived next door to me. Instead of hauling myself across town to the hospital for my weekly massage, the massage came to me. I saw this as another sign that God had not forgotten about me and was in control.

The one question I got the most during this time was, "Are you depressed? We have pills for that."

I wasn't dancing through the streets; don't get me wrong. Dying isn't for the weak. But I had a healthy outlook on death and dying. It's a natural part of life, and I had acknowledged its arrival. My anger had dissipated and was replaced with a calmness. I had arrived at the acceptance phase. Plus, the last thing I needed was more drugs.

At that point, I was unable to walk from my bed to the bathroom without gasping for air. It was a clear indication intervention was needed. The palliative care doctor insisted I use an oxygen tank because my breathing would get worse and she wanted to avoid admitting me to the hospital for full-time breathing assistance.

I didn't like the thought of being on an oxygen tank. It was an outward symbol of my illness, another part of this disease I had to carry, quite literally, while fighting to maintain some semblance of a life. And it was a reminder that my body was not working as it should and would continue to worsen. I acquiesced, however. The tank was better than the hospital, and I ended up using it for many months.

Regardless of my acceptance, some things still had not changed. I shared a converted studio apartment with a roommate who had no idea I had cancer. My hair had grown back, and outwardly, there were few signs I was anything but a pale New Yorker who spent too much time indoors. When she went to work each day, I simply hung around the apartment. When she questioned the noise the oxygen tank made at night, I told her it was a humidifier.

I was good, perhaps too good, at weaving a tale for the people in my life. I kept the two parts of my identity as wholly separate as possible, much like superheroes maintain a low-key façade to protect their alter egos. I didn't want to be treated like a cancer patient.

Then one day I had to wheel the oxygen tank across the living room while she was there visiting with her mom.

"What is that?" she asked, a little incredulous that something that big would fit in our tiny apartment. I ended up coming clean with her. Like others, she was surprised.

Worse than giving in to the oxygen tank was making an appointment to visit a hospice center. Out of all the things I had to do in the course of my illness, that was the most harrowing. In my mind, hospice was for people at the ends of their lives, and until that moment, it had not set in—I was one of those people. I was able to push past the realization that I was dying, that I needed blood transfusions or to use an oxygen tank, but once I was in the hospice center, I felt at the ripe age of twenty-seven my fate was sealed.

One thing that did help me through this somber time was reading *Man's Search for Meaning*. This 1946 book by Viktor Frankl chronicles his experiences as a prisoner in Nazi concentration camps during World War II. He describes his psychotherapeutic method, which involves identifying a purpose in life to feel positive about, and then actively imagining that outcome in the future. According to Frankl, man's deepest desire is to search for meaning and purpose. He believes the way a prisoner—specifically himself—imagines the future affects his longevity; finding his purpose in the aftermath of the Holocaust ultimately was Frankl's reason for his survival of it.

Like Frankl, I'd searched for meaning to everything—life, death, illness, faith—and after reading his book, I realized my purpose for surviving cancer so many times would be fulfilled. While my purpose was not exactly clear to me in that moment, I was confident God had a plan.

There were days I had to dig my nails into my faith and hold on because I'd get mad that I was in my twenties and not likely to see many more years. I had to sort through a lot of emotion to find the peace of mind I'd used to tell my parents and sister my decision to stop treatment.

Prayer certainly played a major part in my life at this time, but I won't tell you I had an epiphany about God's purpose for me. Rather than lift me from the darkness I'd spiraled into, prayer and faith kept me standing against the raging tempest. Sometimes I guess that's the best we can hope for.

And I binge-watched episodes of *Six Feet Under*. I was in a dark, brooding mood. I was obsessed with death. I wasn't looking forward to it, but I was preparing, doing research almost. It's not like I could interview people, so I wanted to see and read as much about the concept of death as I could find. *Six Feet Under* was about the interpretation of death from a variety of viewpoints and what the afterlife would look like.

I also saw a cardiologist.

"You have heart failure due to cardiomyopathy," she told me in a voice that could have belonged to a hundred other doctors I'd talked to over the years. "Excessive amounts of radiation and one of the chemo agents, Adriamycin, from your ABVD treatment likely caused the weakening of heart muscles."

"The gift that never stops giving," I deadpanned.

Ignoring my attempt at sarcasm, she misdiagnosed me with reversible heart damage and put me on oxygen. Then I saw a pulmonologist who said the previous diagnosis of asthma was incorrect and that my pulmonary fibrosis was secondary to radiation toxicity and not Bleomycin toxicity. Radiation toxicity can be reversed, but it's made worse by oxygen.

Does anyone wonder why I question the health care profession so much?

As I weaned myself off the oxygen, I began to feel better. I'd had a wish to live in Spain since AP Spanish in high school, so I decided to plan a trip. I'd read a story about an American girl living in Seville, sitting at a tapas bar, sharing a glass of wine with friends. I always envisioned that girl would be me someday, and I was going to make it happen.

I left three days after my sister's wedding in November. I knew I had, at most, a year to live, so I spent my entire life savings on the trip. There was no future to plan for—certainly no wedding in my future, no retirement to worry about. My time was now, and I was going to live every moment.

When I got to Seville, I shared a house with three English-speaking travelers. The homeowner and his brother had an Irish bar in the main village center and ran a college exchange program. There was access to a lot of international students, which worked out well because they were always up for exploring neighboring cities and taking overnight trips.

I was a carefree twenty-something New Yorker living a virtually stress-free life in Spain. No one knew about my illness. I could be whoever I wanted to be. I told those around me the version of my life I chose and liked. I lived on the Spanish diet of small meals throughout the day and a siesta in the afternoon. I was not ingesting foods that were genetically modified or injected with hormones.

And Spain was absolutely beautiful, so I walked everywhere beneath the blue skies and temperate weather. The longer I was there, the more I saw my lung and heart capacity increase. I had gone to Spain to die, but every day, I felt more alive.

I realized God had created my body with an intuition and ability, and when left alone, it had the power to heal itself. Listening to that intuition in New York, I'd left behind the toxicity of chemo and radiation and drugs meant to help me fight for my life, but all it had done was weaken me in body and spirit.

While in Seville, I met a Dutch girl named Nina who was doing a semester abroad in Seville. We instantly clicked. Nina and I took day trips exploring the countryside, visiting museums and galleries, whatever appealed to us. In the evenings we would visit the tapas bars and dance the night away. I became the girl of my dreams, sharing a glass of wine with a friend. Fluent in Spanish, Nina often acted as my translator. Later she would become a bigger part of my life, but while in Seville, I was never able to open up to her about my health issues. Old habits die hard, I guess.

I spent a total of three months in Spain and enjoyed every moment of it. Ironically, I was only getting stronger and healthier, so I decided it was time to come back home.

CHAPTER 20

No Support Group for You

I returned from my trip in January 2008 and spent the next few months stuck in a weird routine where I would wake up and my first thought would be, "Okay, I am not dead yet. What should I do to kill time today?"

While abroad, I'd created an identity of a competent lawyer at the top of her game. But now, I had nothing but time on my hands. I needed to keep myself busy to avoid thinking about slowly dying.

Up to this point, I had felt it was important to be around people who knew nothing about what I was going through. The majority of my family still didn't know the truth of my diagnosis or prognosis, as my parents had kept it a secret. They still hadn't told the family about Loren's diagnosis and she'd been cancer-free for years.

I didn't want the specter of my prognosis constantly hanging over me through the pitying looks and well-meaning questions of people, nor did I want to repeat the same sad story over and over. And I could get away with it. I didn't look like someone with terminal cancer. I looked like a fit, dark-haired woman in the peak of health and vibrancy, living her life, meeting men and taking on the world.

It was a really good disguise as disguises go.

But it wasn't me—not the real me—and I felt I couldn't run from the truth any longer. Not telling anyone about my cancer for so long ingrained a terrible feeling of shame in me. It left me isolated and alone, so it was hard opening up. In some ways, I felt guilty about laying the burden of my illness on another person's shoulders. By keeping it a secret, I kept the weight solely where I thought it belonged. But then it began to feel like a punishment, and I knew it was time to reach out for help.

I began searching for support groups for people with cancer. I thought it would be helpful to spend time with people who were going through what I was. Shared journeys, shared pain, right? Maybe I would find answers to some of my questions by listening to them talk about their own experiences. But there's something interesting about having cancer in your twenties. No one expects you to look healthy and young when you're dying of cancer.

I remember walking into one group of people with terminal cancer and almost everyone was between sixty and eighty years old; some were even older. I walked inside the room and every head turned my way.

"Can I help you?" A middle-aged woman left the circle of folding chairs and approached, her hands clasped in front of her body. Her brows were drawn together into a single line over the bridge of her nose, as if she were unused to seeing people walk into the room.

"I'm here for the cancer support group." I gave her a weak smile. Did I sound apologetic? Why should I be apologizing? I was the one with cancer.

She looked over my shoulder and I followed her gaze. "Are you meeting someone? A parent or grandparent maybe?"

"No, just me. I got the group name from my oncologist's office."

Her face morphed from the scrunched caterpillar into a wide-eyed kewpie doll, with her mouth making the full "o" of surprise. Behind her, heads started to swivel away. Hushed whispers. Slow nods and pitied looks were shared as if I couldn't see or hear them.

It took me a minute to realize the source of the weird look on her face and the faces around the room; I didn't look like someone with terminal cancer. I was too young. Too healthy looking. Too alive.

I defied all of their assumptions about death and dying.

Okay, I thought, *no more grandma and grandpa clubs.*

I tried again, finding a support group for cancer patients in their twenties, but that didn't go any better. The unspoken reality was that the groups for young people were all about *surviving* cancer, not dying from it. Since my cancer had come back several times, my journey scared them even more. They wanted to be cured and move on with their lives. Just like my friend Wael in California had been afraid for me to share my story with his daughter, they saw me as a reminder that being cured might not happen. Or worse, you could be cured and fall ill again.

I could sympathize with them. To deal with your own mortality alone in a dark bedroom is one thing. But to have it sit in front of you in a place you came to for hope, that's more than most people can bear. I was the villain in their story, however unintentional my role. I was the thing they feared, the monster in the closet. Before the end of the first meeting, I slipped out quietly and never returned.

After those two failed attempts, I found a place called Gilda's Club. It was founded by the actor, Gene Wilder, in memory of his late wife, Gilda Radner. She had passed in 1989 from ovarian cancer, and Gilda's Clubs were started all over the United States to support cancer patients, their families, and friends.

Gilda's Club quickly became a refuge for me, much like dating had been. I felt free to express myself there and loved the activities they offered: art classes, yoga and meditation, and support groups of various kinds. I could share my story or not. I could be Rinad the Twenty-Something Lawyer or Rinad the Cancer Patient with a terminal diagnosis, or just Rinad. My identity was as fluid as the days of the week.

But even in Gilda's Club, the feeling of support eventually wore thin. Many of the participants looked at me with an attitude that seemed to say, "Why are you here? You look too young and healthy to have terminal cancer." Again, I could sympathize. After all, I was running around the city on dates, I had all my hair, and I looked great.

I didn't look like I was dying.

One day in the support group, the anger was boiling over about what I was going through. From the initial diagnosis of "that cancer is the easiest to deal with," I'd expected my treatment and cure to be as straightforward as my sister's treatment had been. Cancer would be just another test I would ace because I would follow the rules.

On that day, all of my stupid, short-sighted expectations came crashing down. I'd ignored my instincts time and time again. I'd listened to doctors, one after the other, when their diagnoses were proven incorrect, even when their treatments nearly killed me. I was second-guessing every decision I had ever made. The emotions crashed in on me like the proverbial tidal wave. I began crying and cursing so loudly and aggressively that I got kicked out of Gilda's Club.

I agonized about how ten years earlier I had never had any trouble getting into clubs when I was in college. Every weekend, my friends and I would head to Babylon, The Bank, or Pangea in downtown DC and dance the night away. It was our ritual, and I always felt like a VIP. The bouncers and regulars all knew me, and my friends and I would skip the line and walk right in on cold winter nights. I guess you could say I was used to being admitted wherever I wanted to go.

Now, even a club for cancer patients didn't want me.

Could it get any lower than that?

CHAPTER 21

Don't Put Dirt on My Grave Just Yet

Day after day, week after week, all the peace I had felt letting go of treatment and control had worn off. I was starting to get really annoyed that the end had not yet come. Now that's a strange conversation to have with God in your nightly prayers. The song by *Nashville* kept playing through my head: "Don't put dirt on my grave just yet."

I wasn't dead. What's worse, I was getting stronger. I had spent all my savings on a bucket list trip thinking I didn't need a savings account. Now, I was a law-school graduate, an attorney with no license, no job, and no money with tons of school debt.

I'd finally started breaking the rules and look where it had gotten me. An unknown future. To me, that was much more terrifying than death.

I was handling operations for my brother's mortgage company in exchange for him paying my rent, but that took a minimal amount of my time. His generosity really had made my *life* possible, and I couldn't appreciate him more for it.

But I needed to do something with my life, and if I wasn't going to die, I needed to figure out what that was.

When I returned from Spain, I took a trip with Jeanne to a monastery upstate to help me de-stress. I thought spending some time in silence, meditating, would give me some much-needed clarity. But there were *challenges*.

First, it was a vegan environment, and I needed heavy proteins like eggs, cheese, red meat, and fish to keep my red blood cell count up. On top of that, it was the middle of winter in northern New York and there wasn't adequate heat. So, instead of a state of clarity, I got to be dizzy, weak, and freezing. Jeanne ended up carrying me around the campus all weekend.

✝

"Rinad, you have to have faith. You have to really believe and it will come true."

No, Jeanne wasn't talking about a cure; she was referring to the upcoming Super Bowl game I planned to watch that night where my beloved team, the New York Giants, were slated to play the undefeated Patriots. The Giants were picked to lose. Even so, I don't know what excited me more: the chance at the trophy or to eat a cheeseburger. And believe I did, willing the Giants to their victory. While I was out with friends that night, my wallet was stolen, which put a damper on the festivities. What a way to take the brand-new wind out of my tattered sails.

However, this turned out to be a blessing in disguise. I was forced to get new insurance cards and, in the process, learned that my plan had changed. Now, some super-reputable doctors were in my network. I immediately made appointments to see a top-rated oncologist and cardiologist.

The oncologist I chose, Dr. L, was stern and not at all personable, and to make matters worse, incredibly arrogant. His prognosis, however, was consistent with my last oncologist—not in terms of the timeline, as I clearly was nowhere near dead eleven months after the six-month pronouncement of my demise.

He offered me the same chemo and blood transfusion maintenance protocol but said there was no way to cure me without a bone marrow transplant that my heart and lungs could not tolerate. I declined all options, and he told me I had no more than two years left. This would have me expiring in May 2010. I crossed my fingers, thanked him for his time, and never went back.

The new cardiologist disagreed with much of what the previous one had said. This was a constant battle in my journey toward treatment, if not a cure. Doctors often give *opinions*. Medicine is a *practice*. How is an untrained patient supposed to filter through the complicated information and make an informed decision without going to medical school?

Basically, the new cardiologist said there was no guarantee I would get better, even if I took medication for years. My echo actually showed a worsening result, so I immediately stopped taking the meds I was on because they were making me feel dizzy and light-headed. I learned later that alternative medications existed that would have potentially offered the same benefits as the medicine I was taking without making me feel so bad. However, neither cardiologist I saw had specialized in cardiomyopathy due to secondary chemo and radiation poisoning, so neither had known to advise me on that protocol. Had I been taking the right meds from 2008 to 2010, I might have prevented damage to my heart and would likely have restored some of my heart function. This was valuable time I did not have to waste.

During the summer of 2008, my Dutch friend from Seville, Nina, came to visit me in New York. Wanting to avoid any more deception, I finally told her of all my health issues and confessed to why I had taken the trip to Seville. She was shocked, saying the same things most people did when they found out—it was amazing I could be suffering from such ailments and not look or act sick. And like others before her, she surprised me with her acceptance. She didn't run, and she wasn't angry at my having lied to her. We just did our best to treat each other normally.

We enjoyed our time together in New York City, living it up as only two young women in their twenties can. One night at a happy hour at Tavern on the Green, we met two friends named Chris and Steve. Steve was instantly attracted to Nina, and they struck up a conversation, which left me with Chris.

Chris was handsome, funny, smart . . . all tic marks on the boyfriend checklist, but despite his best attempts at flirting, I wasn't initially into him. When Nina and Steve abandoned us for another party in the Meatpacking District, Chris dragged me into a cab for the trek downtown. He was quick-witted and charming, and maybe it was the hours of drinks and the intimate atmosphere of a nighttime ride across town staring at the big city lights that started to change how I saw him.

I suddenly confessed, "I have cancer." The words were heavy in the dark interior of the cab. I think I heard the driver gasp, but Chris, to his credit, didn't react. "I'm in a weird limbo right now. Not really remission but feeling good."

He grinned. It was a look full of promise and interest and all the things a woman wants to see on a man's face. "Feeling good sounds like a reason to enjoy the evening and worry about tomorrow at another time."

We met up with Nina and Steve and later went out to dinner. It was one of those nights everyone is entitled to in life: perfect. We laughed, ate good food, had too many drinks, and I poured myself into bed just as the sun was coming up.

Chris and I ended up having a lot in common. We all made plans to spend the next day on Chris' boat docked in Sag Harbor. He made quite the dashing captain! The four of us spent the weekends that summer in the Hamptons. Nina and I would grab the Jitney on Friday and we'd live it up with Chris and Steve on the boat or beach or just hanging out in her Hamptons summer rental. It's amazing what the right bathing suit or lighting can do to hide blemishes or surgical scars. On Sunday, we'd take the Jitney home again. I finally felt like a single girl living in the Big Apple and having the encounters normal twenty-somethings should have. I'd like to think I made Carrie Bradshaw proud.

Chris didn't ask questions about my midnight taxi confession, and I didn't offer any further details. Cabs in New York after midnight are a lot like Las Vegas—what happens there, stays there. It was a great summer, but in my life, great things like that didn't tend to last.

While on the Jet Ski one afternoon, I started feeling a weird pain in my hips. It would crop up and go away, then come back stronger each time. At one point, my right hip completely locked and fear slipped in. How was I going to explain this to everyone? I didn't want to ruin the party. When I returned to the city, walking around on the hard pavement exacerbated the pain. It got so bad I couldn't ignore it any longer.

I got a PET scan that August and learned the cancer had spread to my right hip.

Life #5

CHAPTER 22

If I'm Careful

That Monday morning, I was referred to an orthopedic surgeon, who referred me to a new radiation oncologist. Being back in that position made me angry because I had sworn off all treatments for cancer back in June 2007 and was adamantly against more radiation. But looking on the bright side, this time around I was at a very reputable hospital in mid-town Manhattan with top-grade machines, thanks to getting my wallet stolen.

"You're a lawyer, Ms. Bsharat." The doctor tried to reason with me after I vehemently opposed his prescribed treatment. "Surely you can see the value in a plea deal."

I hesitated for a moment, curious. Doctors had rarely tried to reason with me, usually choosing to ignore or overrule me. "What's your offer then?"

"Radiation is the lesser of two evils. Without it, the cancer will weaken your bones, and if you fall, you'll likely break your hip. That would require a hip replacement. Mending the hip with surgery would be a six-month to one-year recovery period, which is time you don't have. Whereas radiation would only take two weeks."

As arguments go, it was fairly sound. So, with a lot of hesitancy, I reversed course and decided to pursue radiation therapy for the cancer in my hip. I wanted to live out my last days as comfortably as possible and that involved walking. This option was not going to cure the cancer, but it would increase my standard of living.

The radiation oncologist repeated everything the surgeon had said with a curious caveat. "If I'm careful, I can avoid the ovaries."

He wasn't joking.

"What do you mean 'if you are careful'?"

He backtracked immediately. "I'm sorry. It was a poor choice of words."

But by then, the damage to my already fragile confidence was done. What did I need ovaries for? I would be dead in a couple of years at most, the option of having children was already out the window, another side effect of the MVP back in 2005. I would rather have working hips, so I moved forward with the radiation treatments. But the decision to avoid treatment wasn't the only thing I went back on.

The real issue was that I started to lose faith that I would be dead soon. It was dragging out, month after month, and frankly, I was terrified—not about death, I had come to terms with that. I expected it. I was terrified at the prospect before me of living for some indeterminate amount of time. And without a plan or savings!

It was now more than a year after my initial prognosis from Dr. L. I had blown all of my money on what I thought was going to be my swan song in Spain. Now, I had to find some way to give my remaining time some kind of meaning. I needed a purpose, something to fixate on, other than my impending-but-never-occurring death.

Back when I'd reversed course about medical school, I'd relied on a message in a dream to steer me toward law school. God's subtle voice came to me in a similar fashion a second time around. This time, I dreamed I was a judge standing before a great brick wall, and behind that wall stood thousands of patients all waiting on a treatment or cure. With each crack of my gavel, I removed one brick in the wall.

I wasn't vain enough to think I could deliver anyone a cure, but maybe I could help get rid of some obstacles through the law. I'd become a lawyer with the hopes of using my degree in health care law.

So, in November 2008, I decided it was time to study for the bar exam.

When I spoke to my parents, they supported me 100 percent. They agreed to give me rent money every month while I studied since I would not have time to consult for my brother's firm. The BAR/BRI class started on December 18, the day after my twenty-ninth birthday.

My parents did have some concerns, however. Knowing I was ultra-competitive and always had to get the highest grade in class, they worried I would create undue stress my body couldn't handle. I made a deal with them. I would approach the test on my first attempt like it was a practice exam.

While I studied my butt off every day for two months, I tried to look at it like a rehearsal for the real thing. But I had no idea how to do that. Doing something halfway is not a thing that exists anywhere in my nature. Perfectionism exists in my make-up. Persistence. The inability to let opportunities pass me by. Those are second nature. My time was short, and I was determined to make the most of it.

Rather than see it as a detriment to my health, I believe it was what Frankl described in his book: I saw it as my purpose. There was a reason I woke up every morning.

I made a study schedule that I stuck to every day. Every morning after breakfast, I went to Fordham Law Library to study. I would study for four hours, then take a lunch break. After that, I studied again until 6 p.m., went home, ate dinner, and studied again until ten at night. I did this every day, six days a week, until the day of the exam on February 28.

I should also mention that during this time, my ebb and flow relationship with God was trending in a positive direction. I still prayed constantly for strength and kept an open line to God asking for guidance, or mainly to ask Him, *What are you thinking?* But it was still something that I pulled out when I was frightened or in need. I was not strong in it yet.

In 2008, I reconnected with my youth pastor from childhood, Pastor Joey. We'd lost contact when he accepted a position at a different church when I was fifteen, and I was excited to hear he was pastoring a church ten blocks away from where I lived. I looked forward to reconnecting with him.

What I didn't know was that I would also be connecting with God on a level I had never experienced before.

It was an informal church that met in an off-Broadway theater in the upper west side above a Turkish restaurant. When you walked in, coffee and donuts were waiting for you. Everyone wore jeans and there was a rock band. This was a sharp contrast to the formal church of my youth. My first thought was, *This is how I need to do church.*

Joey and the lead pastor prayed with me in the back room, and that began my journey of returning to a relationship with God. Pastor Joey and I met for weekly prayer sessions for several months. I was still angry about my health, but I also felt like I was having another wave of revelation about God and His love for me, as I read in *The Shack.*

I went to church every week. I was drawn there in a way I had never been. When they prayed for me, I felt my spirit move, like I had awakened, and my senses were sharper. Joey also introduced me to a girl named Won, who had just passed the New York bar exam. She had grown up in a Korean household, and although she was a few years younger than me, her faith was much stronger than mine.

The curious, inquisitive part of me started asking questions, and I did not hold back. Not only was I completely in awe that Won had just slayed the dragon of the bar exam that I'd been dreading for three years, but she also had this confidence that stretched beyond knowledge of the law. She knew exactly who she was, and where her relationship with God stood.

I didn't realize it until then, but my relationship with God was very one-dimensional. Yes, I had faith. But it was the faith of a person who reached out for the life preserver when they were drowning. When you're drowning, you'll reach for anything.

We spoke about our experiences and upbringing, and she would quote Scripture and relate the passages back to her life. I wanted to be at a point where I could do that, where I *wanted* to do that. I could quote regulations in law, but I wanted to have that same understanding of the Bible.

Won ended up giving me her bar study outline, which had been passed around Columbia Law School. I followed it to the letter. After the exam, I felt on top of the world. I was physically and emotionally drained, but proud to have taken this monumental step. Just like with law school, if I failed while trying, at least I would have no regrets.

But just like law school, I didn't fail.

When I found out I passed, I felt like my professional options were endless, that maybe it wasn't the end of the road for me. Not yet at least. Bisseh still had a few lives left to live.

And Won had opened my mind to new thoughts about my relationship with God. What I had read in *The Shack*, she lived out in her life. For the first time in a long time, I was attending church because I enjoyed the worship and the message, not because I had some moral obligation. I had grown up in a Presbyterian church, where we sang hymns from books written in the 1900s, accompanied by an organ. It was conservative in both the liturgy and the attire. When I started going to Pastor Joey's church, I saw how animated worship could be. I learned that you could wear jeans and rock out on drums and still be praising God.

I was living my life with renewed purpose and fighting every day. By May 2009, I had lived one year out of the two that Dr. L had predicted I had left. Each day was a struggle, but I was starting to accept it. There were times when I even felt my way of living was normal. This had a lot to do with Pastor Joey's church and my reconnection with God. I had become more thankful than resentful.

It was starting to affect my health.

I'd not felt this good in five years. I was almost scared to use the word, but I felt hopeful.

After I got my bar results, I thought a lot about what my dream job would be. The answer came one day randomly while I was getting a pedicure. I overheard a woman telling a story about her husband and how he'd lost his job and health insurance benefits and now couldn't get insurance to cover his treatment for some condition because it was considered pre-existing. I thought of my own situation after college, and how I'd faced much the same problem when I was returning from the Contiki tour, afraid to go to the doctor and find out I was sick before the insurance kicked in. And that was when I realized where my future waited.

I wanted to help change the health care system.

I wanted to help abolish the concept of pre-existing conditions. I wanted every American to have access to affordable health care. I would help someone else avoid the dreadful experience I had endured for the past five years. And I knew exactly how to do it.

CHAPTER 23

Dr. Death

By mid-2009, with more than half a decade of less-than-desirable experiences with the health community and a passed bar exam in my quiver, I moved forward with my goals to help change the medical industry to provide affordable health care for all.

Through a mutual friend, I had a contact who worked on Capitol Hill. I made the call on a Wednesday in mid-May, interviewed, and by the following week, was offered a position to work on Capitol Hill in the office of Congressman Ed Towns, a Democrat from Brooklyn, New York. I immediately jumped on the opportunity, even though I might not get better anytime soon.

I was sworn into the New York State Appellate Division Second Department on June 8, 2009. Three years after my law school graduation, I was finally an esquire—a licensed attorney! My family rallied behind me in the courtroom as I took the oath. Even Aunt Ellen surprised me and flew up from Virginia to witness this momentous event.

A week later, I moved all of my belongings by train to Washington, DC. It was a little disheartening that after almost thirty years on this planet, everything I owned fit neatly into two large suitcases. Everyone around me was getting married, buying homes, and starting families, while I was moving to Washington, DC, with barely more than the clothes on my back. That was my reality.

The first thing I did was look for a church. I had formed such a close connection with God and, while it may sound crazy, I felt my health improving since I had returned to church, ever since Pastor Joey prayed over me in the back room of the dodgy off-Broadway theater above the Turkish restaurant. He put me in touch with the National Community Church (NCC) in DC. It was the same casual atmosphere—rock band, coffee and donuts served every Sunday—so I became a regular attendee.

My first "home" in Washington, DC, was a long-term house-sitting job near Falls Church. I didn't have a car so I needed easy access to public transportation. From the apartment, however, I could walk to the bus station and then catch the metro downtown. All total, the commute took ninety minutes each way. I often worked ridiculously long days, and if I left even three to five minutes late, I would miss the connection between the metro and bus. Of course, my first month there, it rained for thirty days straight! But rain is certainly easier to deal with than snow and ice.

During that time, I settled into my new job on Capitol Hill. It was incredibly interesting and just what I had envisioned myself doing. After a short stint in Congressman Towns' office, I moved to the House Committee on Oversight and Government Reform, the main investigative committee in the US House of Representatives, where Congressman Towns was the Chairman, which has jurisdiction over health care issues. I was thrilled to be a part of the history-making work on the Hill while the Affordable Care Act, also known as "Obamacare," was being signed into law. This was truly the start of the culmination of my dreams. Although I didn't work on the Care Act specifically, I attended the debates and watched the members of Congress tirelessly work until all hours of the night to pass this legislation in their private chambers.

While I was deeply passionate about the work, I still played my cards close to my chest. I told people I had a sister who'd fought cancer in college and how the wait for her to be added to our mom's insurance almost had devastating effects. I felt less guilty about the little white lie— it was mostly true, after all, just not all for my sister.

But they recognized the fuel for my passion. Health care is a fundamental right. A family shouldn't have to go bankrupt to save their child or decide between feeding the family or filling a prescription. I worked on a variety of health care-related hearings and investigations. During the H1N1 crisis, I was part of the group asking why the pharmaceutical companies didn't have a vaccine and why any vaccines available were going overseas instead of staying in the United States. I also assisted in the investigation on the CEOs of insurance companies making tens of millions in salaries and bonuses, but denying patients' claims.

In September 2009, I moved to my own apartment in Clarendon on the outskirts of Washington, DC. I loved that place, but still had to take the bus and metro to work. I had my eyes on an apartment downtown and put my name on the waiting list. Every day, I would walk by it and pray for my name to be called.

Everything seemed to be going as well as it could in my life, but the peak came in October 2009 when my latest PET scan showed remarkable improvement. The masses up and down my mediastinum had shrunk considerably, causing the doctors to believe the masses in that area were inflammation rather than cancer. The mass in my right lung had also shrunk from 11 cm to around 2.3 cm. I wasn't even on any treatment. I had left my body and immune system alone to do its work, and it was proving to be a good decision.

More than that, however. I had put my faith where it needed to be, and God was showing me the choice was a good one. My mantra of *take me or heal me* was being answered, this time on the side of healing. I wasn't cured and I knew that. But in body and spirit, I felt as whole as I had for a long time. My focus, as it had been when I was younger before the cancer had become the center of my universe, was on learning and hard work.

I still battled the loneliness, but for the first time, I didn't feel alone. I knew God was with me.

Full of the confidence that comes from improved health and life's goals unfolding, the next month I met Karl at a house party. Having learned positive lessons from Ajay, Harold, and Chris, I was completely open with Karl from the beginning. For the first time in my journey, I saw hope and wasn't afraid of the future . . . or of sharing it.

One drawback of looking perfectly healthy, however, was that people take for granted you are perfectly healthy. On our third date, Karl planned a surprise. I dressed for a night out—flirty little red dress, kitten heels, full makeup—but I didn't really know anything about the evening he had planned until we arrived at the parking lot of the stadium, packed to the brim with cars, limousines, and buses. He'd gotten third row tickets to a U2 concert! We ended up having to park about a mile from the venue, and walking in heels with one lung and half a heart did not sit well with me. I was exhausted and sweating by the time we sat down. Twenty minutes later, however, Nancy Pelosi and her bodyguard sat down right behind us, so the night was interesting to say the least.

Karl was a serious athlete, training for marathons and triathlons throughout our relationship, and he motivated me to get serious about working out as well. Up until then, I was always on the thin side. But when I hit my thirties, my metabolism slowed way down. Suddenly, I had to pay attention to what I ate and—dare I say it—count my calories. The walk to the concert also proved to me I needed to build up my heart and lung function as much as possible.

For the first time, I joined a gym for weight loss and not just for the social aspect. I was hesitant about physical exercise at first, since I was still very short of breath due to the pulmonary and cardiology problems. The heart is a muscle and needs to be conditioned, the trainers told me, and cardio workouts, however painful or uncomfortable, could help strengthen whatever muscle was not permanently damaged.

Karl helped me develop a good workout routine that took into account my health limitations but didn't treat me like a sick person. He wanted to make me sweat!

I was also sweating out the wait on news about a new job. At the beginning of February 2010, I got an interview for a position at the Department of Justice, and the following month, found out I had gotten the job. The Department of Justice is two blocks from the White House, directly across the street from the apartment I had been eyeing for about six months. I visited the property manager every week asking for vacancies, and received notice shortly after I got the job that the apartment was mine. Once again, the Universe was showing me persistence did pay off!

Memorial Day weekend, I traveled to North Carolina to meet up with my college friends and randomly met a cardiology resident at a house party.

As you know by now, I don't believe in coincidences, but divine interventions, and I saw this chance occurrence as another in a long string of *right place, right time* moments: meeting Wael, the massage therapist living next door, finding the book, *The Shack*. This encounter would be another of those moments for me.

I took the opportunity to chew his ear off and explained my heart problems in excruciating detail. He told me that since my cardiomyopathy was related to chemo and radiation poisoning, I would need to take drugs that worked like Coreg and Altace—the drugs the doctor in New York had prescribed—but had the added benefit of not lowering my blood pressure. Who would have known that combination existed? He found me a doctor in Washington, DC, with the appropriate experience, and I quickly made an appointment.

Though my history with doctors had not been the most pleasant to this point, I immediately trusted Dr. N. He redid the echo test, which showed I was back in heart failure. I had always been in a constant state of shortness of breath, whether it was the chemo, cancer in or around the lung, or the pulmonary fibrosis. Every time I complained to my oncologist, pulmonologist, or cardiologist, they would point to either of these ailments individually or blame them collectively as the culprit. So, I learned to live with it. I made changes to my lifestyle and became immobile. I took a cab everywhere and stayed within a two-block radius if I needed to walk. I lived across the street from work, so that helped. Up until then, there was never any way to decide what ailment was causing the breathing trouble.

My heart then took center stage. My ejection fraction was at an all-time low of 17 percent—dangerous heart transplant territory. He also told me my heart only had about ten years left. It was the first time I knew for sure my heart could be the cause of my demise. It had always been the cancer I had to be wary of, but now I had a second reason to fear.

I'd stopped taking the heart medication because it made me feel dizzy, light-headed, and nauseous. Dr. N told me there was no way to undo the damage already done, but he could prevent further damage by starting the new drugs. In addition, he urged me to have a defibrillator surgically implanted to automatically restart my heart in case it stopped beating.

I was feeling good for the most part. My life was moving forward with work and with Karl. I'd rediscovered my passion for life while living in Washington, DC. Getting the defibrillator, however medically sound it may have been, felt like a step back toward the old Rinad. The sick Rinad. Rinad, the Cancer Patient. So, I refused. If my heart stopped beating, God would either start it up again or call me home.

And there was one other big concern Dr. N dropped like a bomb in my life. The damage to my lung was so extensive that I would need a dual heart and lung transplant within five to ten years. After the transplant, I would be on antirejection medications for the rest of my life, which would lower my immune system and could even cause . . . Hodgkin's Lymphoma. The irony! To be eligible for the transplant, I would need to be in remission for five years, which I knew would be impossible. I decided to placate Dr. N by seeing an oncologist to confirm where I stood in order to start the remission clock. To be brutally honest, I was placating my curiosity even more.

You know what they say about curiosity? It kills the cat.

Dr. N referred me to an oncologist lymphoma specialist, whom I will dub Dr. Death for the remainder of this story. The reason will soon become obvious. Dr. Death ordered the PET scan and a cold-washing bronchoscopy, which confirmed the presence of lymphoma. The five-year clock could not be started yet.

Dr. Death informed me in terms as cold as his name would suggest: "Your heart is too weak. You will not survive any more chemotherapy. To be honest, you've defied all the odds. There is no medical or scientific reason for you to be alive."

"Just because you can't explain it doesn't mean there's not a reason. Maybe God has a reason and I'm alive because of His will. Maybe we just don't know His purpose yet."

He got angry about my belief that God was sustaining me. "I don't believe in God or miracles, Ms. Bsharat. I've spent my life studying medicine, not philosophy or religion. And my reasoned belief is that you are living on borrowed time. I do not believe your heart will last as it is now. You will not live much longer."

I can understand why he got angry. He didn't believe in God or miracles; they went against what he could concretely study in school or prove with his science. Even allowing the possibility of the miraculous would have created discord in his mind and shaken the foundations of his worldview. That's hard to deal with.

But with his cold delivery of my impending demise . . . he earned the nickname Dr. Death.

Dr. Death was not the first skeptic I'd encountered, and I've always tried to have the perspective that every person is entitled to their own opinion, especially when it comes to God. But I'd like to believe that respect is returned. I did not have a problem with Dr. Death being a nonbeliever. However, mocking me for believing my faith was a force in my life was going a little too far.

After my meeting with Dr. Death, I sent my records to another hospital with the hope they would have new tricks up their sleeve. It was a world-class research center with resources exceeded only by its reputation so it would have a finger on the pulse of new up-and-coming trials the smaller centers wouldn't know about.

A few weeks later, this hospital sent me a letter saying they had no options for me. They refused to even set up an appointment for me to be evaluated. For some reason, maybe because of my newfound confidence or because of all the things I now had going for me, I did not take those events to heart. I knew there was something out there for me. I just needed to be patient and have faith, and the right path would reveal itself.

Dr. N also referred me to a pulmonologist, Dr. B. He was mild-mannered and humble, and I enjoyed sitting with him to discuss my health history. He disagreed with much of what my previous two pulmonologists from New York had said.

He said there was no difference between fibrosis due to radiation therapy and Bleomycin toxicity—both were incurable. He also said I didn't have asthma, that my difficulty breathing was due to the following three factors: the talc cement scars; my right lung being deflated by 30 percent; and a possibility of tumors present. Also, the heart failure could be the main reason for my shortness of breath. Visiting these doctors was like being in a boxing match with both hands tied behind your back. But I was determined not to let all of this bad news stop the daily routine of my life, however short the rest of it might be.

✝

On Labor Day weekend 2010, I went to a conference with the Arabic Baptist Church. I was hesitant at first. Not only was it all in Arabic, and mainly the Egyptian dialect, but I also did not know anyone there. However, I thought back to the trips to Mexico, where I had literally chosen to put my life in the hands of complete strangers. I would not be deterred by a simple church conference!

I am glad I decided to go; it was a turning point in my faith. Some of the people I met became great role models for me, showing me what I wanted to become as a Christian. They were confident in their faith, and that was not something I had ever experienced. I was always questioning: What was my place with God? What was His place with me? Did He really love me unconditionally? I sounded like a love-struck teenage girl.

At this conference, I learned I needed some quiet devotion time every morning before starting my day. My faith was always something I turned to in the hard times. It was a backup plan in a way. By making it a part of my daily routine, I'm able to center my thoughts and emotions with my faith in God's plan for me. In some ways, it's a reminder of the answers to my big question: Why haven't You healed me or taken me? By reminding myself of those answers at the start of my day, I find I am more at peace.

Many people think they can't make time for such devotion, but it's not hard because we have little pockets of space in our day we can fill. I often read the Bible and write in my journal while drinking my coffee first thing in the morning. Then I get ready while listening to Joel Osteen or Joyce Meyer. When I cannot make it to church in person, I listen to the National Community Church or Metro DC sermons online or in podcasts.

Setting aside time every day allows me to live in the moment. When I'm anxious about the future, this devotional time reminds me to have faith and let God provide. I wasn't there yet in terms of my faith, but I wanted to be. I wanted to let go of the regret for the past, remember that God has a plan for me, and not worry about the future. I wanted to enjoy the life I have.

One workshop at the conference was about finding God's will for us. God shows us His plan for us in a million different ways. We just have to be willing to see them for what they are. It was easy to think of my cancer as a punishment, but how many doctors had told me I shouldn't have survived? My survival is God's will. I am here for a purpose, even if I don't always understand it. Or my doctors can't explain it.

It opened my eyes to having God be a part of my day-to-day decision-making process. Never before had I thought the almighty God had time to think about my tedious needs. It's easy to think He has much bigger things to worry about, even if I am fighting for my life. But the opposite is true. We can have direct conversations with God, and He wants us to commune with Him daily. He fills our heart with His love and wisdom if we will only listen.

I met some strong Christians that weekend, some I stayed in touch with for many years. Eva, a young woman from Michigan, had come to Washington, DC for a rotation in medical school and ended up staying with me for three months. She would wake up every morning at 4:30 a.m. and read the Bible for half an hour before walking two miles to work a full day. Working at a DC children's hospital is no easy task, but I saw a force in this young woman as she dealt with the daily horrors of her job. She told me she found strength in knowing she was living up to God's purpose for her and that He would see her through the most difficult time. With that knowledge, she knew she could face anything.

Eva was five years younger than me, but she was a more mature Christian. Like Won had before, her dedication inspired me to become more consistent in my faith. I wanted to *know*, as she did, I was living the right life, not for myself but for God.

During that time, I applied for and received a scholarship from the Leukemia and Lymphoma Society. They paid for insurance premiums and co-pays for prescriptions. This helped my mounting bills tremendously. I also applied for a scholarship with The Samfund, and they assisted with my rent. So many organizations and nonprofits are available for specific needs and disease categories; it is important to look into all resources.

I imagine anyone with a complicated or long-term health crisis gets to a point with medical bills where they either let the weight of the number crush them, or they simply put it aside to think about another day. Your point of view becomes, "I'm alive and breathing and not in the hospital. I hope I'm able to pay for it, but if not, I just don't care." These scholarships helped me keep the worry about medical bills safely tucked away while I focused on more important things: staying healthy and strengthening my faith. This was why I wanted to change the health care system. I had choices, however difficult or poor they might be. Many people do not.

Despite my health woes, things were looking up for me. I had an apartment I loved, great friends, a dream job, a beautiful church family, and to top it all off, I was sworn into the Washington, DC bar in October 2010. I went from no legal licenses to two in a matter of a year.

It was a bittersweet week for me, however.

As I was celebrating my professional accomplishment, I received news that my grandmother, Taita, had passed away. I was unable to rush home because of the swearing-in ceremony, but I did make it home the following week for the funeral.

Taita was the reason our family members were all such strong

Christians. Historically, Christians in the Middle East are of the Catholic or Orthodox faith. But my grandmother felt there was something different.

Her path had crossed with Charles Stanley Ministries. They established a church in Mafraq, and once she heard those pastors preach, she knew they spoke to her with God's voice. She would take two or three of her children to Stanley's church each Sunday without her husband's knowledge because of his strong attachment to the Orthodox church. She put aside the beliefs of Catholicism because of an inner voice, what I called God's nudge, toward a different way of thinking. Taita was very instrumental in choosing her faith and held the belief that these teachings would keep her family safe and healthy. She often prayed blessings over her children and her future grandchildren, planting seeds for future generations.

I didn't know her well, but her legacy was something imprinted on me and future generations because of her faith. She started the journey, and now it was up to me to keep it going.

I was still trying to fully comprehend my relationship with God, working daily on believing that my cancer was not an accident. This belief helped me through the tough times, and it was also helping me through a major non-health trial: being okay with turning thirty and still being single.

Karl and I had broken up. I knew he wasn't right for me, so forcing the relationship and going through the motions was not going to help me find my soulmate. He was a good person— loyal, kind, dependable— but mostly he was convenient. That wasn't fair to either of us. Is it better to be alone or with the wrong person? And why couldn't I find the right person?

I made a conscious decision I would no longer date just for the sake of dating and filling time. I needed to change my mindset. I needed to be okay being alone. I needed to love and feel confident in the new me before I could find meaning in a relationship with another man.

And that would take some time.

Life #6

CHAPTER 24

The Claws Come Out

There are a lot of things you don't know about cancer before you have it: How will your body react to the chemotherapy? How will it feel to tell people, to utter those words, "I have cancer"? No one tells you just how bad that feels. We know pain, we know fatigue, we know what it's like to be sick... but not this sick. This is like a demon inside, greedy in its consumption of you—not just physically, but emotionally and spiritually.

Over time, the physical effects of cancer became apparent. I was weak, constantly out of breath, unable to do the things I always could. The physical limitations were frustrating and annoying. I was a young woman in the prime of my life and wanted to explore and dance and travel.

However, I wasn't prepared for the emotional toll it would take.

I became a version of myself I didn't know and couldn't relate to. I became untrusting, irritable, and controlling. I was like a dog who had been abused and then finally rescued, hesitant at the hands of those trying to help. I believed only I could truly understand what I needed and only I could properly care for me. I developed a short fuse and would blow at a moment's notice and then, frustrated with both those around me and my own behavior, would retreat from the world to recoup. I had been Bisseh, the kitten who grew into the curious and confident cat, exploring the world, walking with surety and poise.

Now I was the caged Tiger.

When you have a health condition, you have to be your own strong advocate. The urgency of your condition will be underestimated, no matter how dire its reputation. Although I did not like seeing who I had to be with health care professionals, this conviction was important to receive the care and treatment I needed. Many times I couldn't control it. Even when completing a mundane task, like buying shoes or calling a plumber, I would have a sense of irrational urgency—a "this must happen now or I will self-destruct" attitude.

The cancer instilled in me the feeling that I would always be deceived or short-changed in some way, particularly when interfacing with doctors. My experiences had not been positive in many aspects, but at the same time, I'd met many wonderful caregivers who wanted to help me. I was, after all, still alive when many had said I would be dead!

Still, I adopted an aggressive, condescending tone. It's perhaps one of my worst traits, and though I'm still working on it, it continues to this day. All scars start with wounds, and if this attitude was my scar, the wound was inflicted at a world-renowned comprehensive cancer center in Washington, DC.

A year after my meeting with Dr. Death, he called out of the blue and informed me that a cancer center was conducting a study on Hodgkin's Lymphoma with an experimental form of chemotherapy that targeted only the Hodgkin's Lymphoma cells. In theory, it would be gentler on the body and prevent hair loss. "But you better decide quick," he warned. "There are limited spaces available and the FDA is looking to close it soon."

I heeded his advice and jumped at the opportunity to enroll.

Guarding access to any health care is the dragon of bureaucracy. Referrals lead to phone calls, which lead to more referrals, which eventually lead to speaking with a secretary, the great gatekeepers of the bureaucracy. I jumped nimbly through each hoop until I was finally told that the person who could connect me with the study gatekeeper, and possibly a cure, was Janet, a new secretary to the department.

I called Janet every day for a week, leaving messages, but she never returned my calls. At last, I called the registration department where she worked and asked someone to physically go to her desk. Finally, I had Janet on the phone. I explained my situation, and the call ended with a simple request: I needed to be seen immediately for the drug trial before it closed.

Before I continue, I want to make something clear: I am not proud of my behavior, but I did what I thought necessary in the fight for my life. I also wish I hadn't had the hope of wellness dangled over my head, like a treat for me to hungrily swipe at, only to have it pulled away without cause or concern.

When you're sick—when you're afraid of dying—you will do anything to stop it, even if you have accepted it. All you want is hope. That's what really keeps you going, and hope is inspired by those who say they can help you. The worst thing is when you know someone can help you and they won't. That makes you an animal, a beast.

A tiger.

Janet didn't get back to me for four days. I even called the front desk and asked the receptionist to leave Janet a written message. Finally, at noon the next day, her voice echoed in my ear, still so sadly apathetic.

"Hello?"

"Yes, hello!" I said. "It's Rinad—"

"I know," she said, interrupting me. "How can I help you?"

Something flared in me, but I forced it down. I needed her. "I'm calling about the appointment with the doctor administering the Brentuximab study, Dr. C. Were you able to get me in with him?"

"Yes, we have you booked for August 31."

This would be the first of many times my heart dropped into my stomach during this conversation.

"August 31, that's . . . that's a month away. I can't—" I stammered.

"It was the first available time the doctor could see you," Janet said, not a hint of anything but indifference and annoyance in her voice. How annoying to have to deal with someone dying.

"There must be something sooner," I pleaded. "Look, I need to see him sooner than that. Really, it's important. I need to be seen while the trial is still open to patients. I know that everyone needs to be seen, I do, but if I could just explain my case more, I think you'd agree—"

"I'm sorry, but there's nothing I can do."

Silence.

I could hear the gates slamming shut on my chances, but I wasn't above begging. "Please, I just visited my cardiologist, and I was diagnosed with Category C heart failure." My voice choked with desperation. I swallowed hard. "I know you know what that means. I haven't been able to find a cure yet, and I don't know how much longer I have."

"I'm sorry, Ms. Bsharat, but there's nothing I can do," she said frigidly.

The conversation ended there.

On August 31, 2011, I went into the office to see Dr. C, the study administrator. Not wanting to waste any more time, I dove into my story of the past fourteen years as soon as he walked into the room.

"Well," Dr. C said as I finished, scribbling on his clipboard and looking between his PA, Sarah, and myself, "you certainly would be an excellent candidate for the SGEN study."

My heart surged. There it was: hope. Already I was reaching for that elusive treat so often dangled before me but never quite within my grasp. I thought my heart might burst with joy.

"Unfortunately," he continued, "the FDA approved the drug a week or so ago, and the study is closed. I'm sorry," he said sanctimoniously. He almost took too much pleasure in delivering my death sentence.

Like a balloon recklessly filled, I burst and saw my hope dissipate into nothingness. My head swam for a moment, then survival mode kicked in.

"I want to do it anyway. Could I start this Friday?" I asked.

He furrowed his brow, confused. Clearly, this was a man who had never had to fight for his life.

"Well . . . " he said, his voice shooting up an octave as he crossed him arms. He considered my chart for a moment. "If you would have been seen prior to the FDA approval date, the pharmaceutical company would have paid for your treatment, but now it's like any other treatment, so you'll have to go through your insurance. Coverage could be spotty, as it usually is with new and expensive treatments like this."

If I had been seen prior to the FDA approval date.

The rage boiled inside of me, pushing at the limits of my composure. Decades of being a passive kitten warred with the tiger scratching to escape. I wanted to go to Janet's desk, and grab her by the collar, and make her look at me, at my history, at what she had done.

"I've been trying to make an appointment for five weeks," I said calmly through my rage.

There was genuine surprise in his eyes. "What?"

I explained my phone calls and lack of response from Janet and he apologized, explaining that Janet was new in the office.

In that moment, a switch flipped.

"I don't care if you're sorry! This is your fault!"

"Ma'am," Dr. C said, "there's no need for you to be abusive. We are dealing with dozens of patients as sick, if not sicker, than you are. We take full responsibility for this mistake."

"Good! You should! This is ridiculous! I did everything I was supposed to do, and now I may die because of your mistake."

"The circumstance is unfortunate, and if we can help—"

"You can administer the drug and wait for a reimbursement!"

I was ranting. I was begging. I was frothing at the mouth. I was a tiger, and my forest was burning down around me.

"The hospital board would never allow that," Dr. C countered, handing me my discharge slip, already heading toward the door.

I crumpled the slip and threw it to the floor. "Then you're not willing to do anything to help, are you? My heart is weakening every day!"

He stared at the crumpled paper, then back at me. "I'm sorry," he said tersely, "but the most I can do is contact your insurance company and appeal to the board for approval to administer the drug before their meeting next month."

Tears welled in my eyes. I felt like ripping my hair out, not a normal instinct for a woman who has been bald as an adult.

That's all I can do.

Those words would prove truer than either of us really knew at that time. Two weeks later, insurance approved the treatment. But Janet requested it as a surgical procedure instead of outpatient chemotherapy administration, so I had to wait another week for that issue to be resolved. After that, it took another five days to squeeze me into the infusion unit. On September 13, 2011, I was given my first dose of the new drug, more than eight weeks after the initial call I made about the trial.

Think about that. At one point, I'd been given three months to live. It took eight weeks, two-thirds of my allotted time left on this planet, to get approved for the treatment I needed to live.

After my first round of chemo, I felt significantly weaker. I couldn't walk from my front door to the elevator, about ten yards, without stopping to catch my breath. Then gradually, the increased exhaustion subsided and I went back to my usual levels of exhaustion. I felt like I was wheezing my way through life, huffing and puffing from one task to the next, from home to work to treatment, and back again.

I went to the DMV and requested a handicap parking decal, then waited almost three weeks before getting a call to tell me the Physician's Certification wasn't filled out properly by Dr. C's office. Another three weeks passed before I was strong enough to get to the DMV and wait four hours in line to correct the mistake.

Fine, I thought. *It's done. I'll let Dr. C know what happened and he can use it as a learning experience for Janet.*

When I went back for another treatment, I explained Janet's mistake, but Dr. C was more focused on questioning my need for the handicap decal.

"Why do you believe you need a handicap placard?"

I was stunned. This was my doctor, the person responsible for my well-being, the one who knew the most about what I was going through medically. How could he be questioning this?

"I have other patients with cancer who don't get a placard. They get by with a walker."

"I know it's easy to forget, sometimes. I look a lot better than I feel. But with the Category C heart failure, I can barely lift my legs, let alone a walker."

He shrugged again and scrawled something on his clipboard. "All right. I guess you know what you need."

Ouch! That's where the conversation ended, but the tone carried over to every interaction that followed. It was hard to breathe in that room with so much of its space taken up by this doctor's giant ego coupled with his ongoing antagonism toward me.

It wasn't the last time he would question my need for disability services. And that's when I realized his lethargy in helping me had nothing to do with a belief that I didn't need assistance. He was punishing me for what he perceived as bad behavior during my initial visit.

I decided to play the game, even though it nearly broke something inside of me. I wasn't wrong to fight for myself and push for treatment and services. But I thought of all the people who would come after me and the power that people like Janet and Dr. C would have over them. I didn't want to be an excuse they used to ignore a plea because "patients could be rude."

I swallowed my pride and apologized to everyone. Some through email, some in person, but each person I had been harsh with received an apology for my behavior. During this visit, Dr. C gave me a hug and told me everything was going to be okay, that I wasn't the first patient who had lashed out *unwarranted* at his staff.

Then he told me, "It's going to be okay; you just have to let the medicine work."

When he said this, something I had been keeping locked up inside burst, and I started to cry . . . hard. I blubbered like a child. Everything I was feeling came out—every feeling of neglect by his staff, every perception of being treated differently because I didn't look like a sick person, all bubbled to the surface. Every appointment, I would come in scared, just wanting to get better, but feeling like nobody cared if I did.

I felt like a teenager again, overwhelmed with emotion with nowhere to put it. This was the one and only time I cried in front of him. He referred me to the chaplain for additional support before my treatment. No more was said of my outburst.

That afternoon, as I was sitting in an armchair, trying to relax with an IV sticking out of my arm, my phone started buzzing. I tried to ignore it at first, but it wouldn't stop. It was a text from one of my cousins.

I am sorry for your loss.

I wrote back, *??*

Our grandfather died.

The phone fell from my hand onto my lap.

It's hard to describe exactly how I felt in that moment. It was a heavy blow. I called my mom to figure out why they hadn't called me to tell me. Her response broke my heart. She didn't want to tell me because she knew I would skip my treatment and rush home. And she was right; I would have dropped everything to be with them. As I sat there with an IV in my arm, completely alone in this treatment center, all I could feel was the grief of my family, hundreds of miles away. I never wanted to be with them more than I did in that moment.

Later that week, I was scheduled for a PET scan. After injecting the radioactive solution, they informed me the machine was broken, something they knew apparently before I even arrived. My health was fragile and consuming the solution once was scary enough; now I would have to do it a second time. Plus I had to take another whole day off work to redo the scan and reschedule my treatment for another day. Neither were things I could afford to do. I explained all of this to an indifferent Dr. C.

As usual, Dr. C had a casual disregard for my concerns, something I should have been used to by this point.

When I asked to be seen in the infusion unit for a round of treatment that day, Dr. C explained how much trouble they'd gone through just to get me scheduled for the following week.

"You should be happy that you got that appointment date at all. We can't just bump you ahead of others and 'squeeze you in' today," he said while making condescending air-quotes.

"You scheduled me for next Thursday?" I asked, exasperated as I looked at the appointment card.

"Yes, it was the soonest available appointment."

My head fell into my hands. "I can't go next Thursday," I explained. "It's my grandfather's memorial service. Why wouldn't you ask for my availability?" I snapped.

He was silent for a moment, flipping through his papers, then looked at me and sighed, "I'm sorry but there's nothing I can do," putting on his best *poor you*-face.

"That seems to be your only response to anything I ask," I snipped.

I was taking the brunt of someone else's mistake, yet again. No matter how I protested, I would be invalidated and ignored and worse, labeled as the problem patient. And yet, I was the one who had to swallow my pride. I was the one dying of cancer, and they had the treatment—the leverage. I had to play their game because Dr. C had already shown himself to be a man willing to punish me for perceived wrongs by withholding services and treatments.

I missed my grandfather's memorial, unable to celebrate his life because I was too busy trying to save my own.

The following week, I brought my father with me to my appointment for support.

"It's going to be okay," Baba said.

I took a deep breath and looked up at the chilly gray DC sky. I folded my arms across my chest and said, "Yeah. Maybe."

After waiting in the lobby for over an hour, we were called in to the examination room. Dr. C finally came in, his face stony and cold. I was ready for a stern talking-to, but not for what he was about to say.

Without preamble, he announced, "Ms. Bsharat, as the head of this division, I have decided we will no longer continue your treatment. Your attitude toward me and my staff has been unacceptable."

I froze. So many thoughts were rushing through my head, but mainly disbelief that this man was going to let me die because he thought

I was rude. I snapped.

"There have been nonstop mistakes by you and your staff, yet my behavior is unacceptable?"

He didn't say anything for a moment. My dark eyes were fixed on his icy blue ones. It was a standoff, and for once, I would not back down. After a lengthy, painful silence, Dr. C was the one to cave.

"We will be ceasing treatment immediately."

I'd stayed with this man after the mounting mistakes and careless attitude because I didn't know my options. But I'd learned a few things over the past year.

"I'm already booked in for an appointment. My insurance has already paid for it. You can't withhold it from me. I'm already here. You must treat me today."

"Ms. Bsharat, I am dropping you as a patient. You will not be treated."

"You're giving me *a death sentence* because of your opinion of my attitude!" I exclaimed. Hot, angry tears were springing up behind my eyes, but I held them back. I wouldn't dare cry in front of this man again. The claws had come out. I felt my father's hand squeeze my shoulder. I'm not sure whether he was agreeing with me or trying to keep me from going full "tiger" on the man across from me.

Reluctantly, Dr. C agreed to administer chemo to me that day. Then, he immediately left the room without doing a medical evaluation or giving any instructions for future treatment. I was left sitting—hands folded in my lap, legs crossed—protecting myself from this place and its people who had made it abundantly clear they didn't care about me or my illness.

He could not be allowed to treat someone like this. The system could not allow him to treat someone like this and get away with it.

"What am I going to do?" I asked, my voice hardly above a whisper, tears pouring freely down my cheeks. I felt another squeeze on my shoulder. Neither my father nor I spoke again until we reached the car.

Neither of us had any words.

Life #7

CHAPTER 25

A Tale of Two Memorial Days

In hindsight, I should have made my departure much sooner from that cancer center. They had proven I was little more than a number or a body to fill an available slot while they billed my insurance company. But it was more than that. They were in the *business* of providing lifesaving treatments and therapies to patients; errors should never be handled lightly. More so, patient concerns should not be dismissed when those errors can literally be the difference between life and death.

I'm an educated person. I went to law school, but I knew little about my options. Because the availability of this treatment was limited by both cost and its experimental nature, it became a competition. Who could get there first rather than who needed it the most became the main criteria for admitting a patient. Couple that with the competitive nature of funding for research, and doctors are often hesitant to take on patients who could adversely impact their statistics.

After my unceremonious exit with Dr. C, I had to scramble to find a new doctor to continue the treatment. I got an appointment with the head of the Lymphoma Department at another facility in Washington, DC. I drove myself to treatments while continuing to work thirty hours a week. I was continuously exhausted, but somehow, I made it through. And because the treatment only targeted the cancerous cells, I didn't lose my hair or blood count, so I never became neutropenic. On February 29, 2012, after nine treatments over twenty-seven weeks, I was finished and, once again, in remission.

The next day, I was on a plane to Greece.

The idea of taking a mission trip with my church came about while I was home recovering from this most recent treatment. I was listening to a podcast on intentional dating and preparing yourself to be ready for Mr. Right (or Ms. Right, as the case may be). One thing recommended was to go on mission trips and volunteer with organizations since you had spare time while still single.

This idea resonated strongly with me because dating was a constant state of conflict. I believe we're meant to do this thing called life in pairs. In my search for a cure to my cancer, I was still searching for a relationship and love. I was desperately lonely for the partnership that comes from being with the right person. Although I knew I was not alone—I had my family and friends, all of whom were very supportive—I wanted to find the person meant to share my life, however long that life might be.

Thus far, I'd dated men who, while kind and sweet in many ways, were not the right men for me. The harder I tried to push each relationship into being the "right" one, the faster it tended to blow up in my face. In some ways, I was at peace with my diagnosis and the very real possibility that I would not be around for a "lifetime" with my future husband. At the same time, I was sticking around longer than expected—in part due to the unending hope of finding my forever someone—and I wanted to find a partner to share the burdens and joys. When relationships didn't work out, I would always console myself by thinking it was better to end it now before it got too serious.

In my early relationships, I did not tell people about the cancer because I didn't want to seem desperate. But I was desperate—desperate for a cure, for love, to figure out my purpose.

As I'd said earlier, cancer is a very selfish disease, but a mission trip was something I could do to give back. Unfortunately, many mission trips are centered around very physical activities: build a school, teach kids to play soccer, or dig a well—none of which I could do—and they also tended to be in remote locations. I had significant health issues to consider and needed to be in a location with US-grade amenities in case I got sick. So, even in my desire to be selfless, I had to be selfish to some degree.

Luckily, my church supported an organization called the A21 Campaign, whose mission was to abolish sexual slavery in the twenty-first century. They provided assistance to human-trafficking survivors.

As someone who had a safe and sheltered childhood, this topic was a difficult reality to be faced with, but I am glad I went. It helped change my perspective about me and what I was dealing with. My worldview had been one of looking inward, only at my own illness, for a long time. I was forced to look outside of my own pain and realize I was not the only person suffering.

Upon returning from Greece, I completed my required three-month follow-up scan, which showed a mass in my left lung that my doctor surmised was just hardened remnants of the pulmonary fibrosis. Everything else was clear, and he would continue to monitor me over time.

I tried to breathe easy.

But it didn't take long before I had my first post-remission scare. Later that month, during Memorial Day weekend 2012, I coughed up about a pint of blood over a six-hour period. I was certain the cancer had returned, but an X-ray showed that the mass had not grown. My lung had collapsed again, due to all the growing and shrinking from previous tumor activity. In November 2012, a follow-up X-ray showed again that I was still in remission.

With the good news, I decided it was time to get my life back on track, and I became more focused on my career.

CHAPTER 26

Déjà Vu

Throughout my sickness, my professional life had been the one thing I always kept moving in the right direction. By this time, I had a resume of working in Congress and at the Department of Justice. I had two law licenses under my belt—I was admitted to the New York State Bar and the District of Columbia Bar. I also served on the board of Christian Legal Aid, providing free assistance to low-income families and individuals regarding landlord-tenant issues or entitlement benefits. My family was doing well; I'd welcomed my first niece into the world.

On the outside, I was your normal thirty-something. Apartment. Job. Friends. Dating. Church. Still, I felt an emptiness in my life. I was constantly receiving invitations to social events for family and friends, all politely addressed to Ms. Rinad Bsharat. Never "Ms. Bsharat and Guest," or "Ms. Bsharat plus one." I went to these events, usually as the only sole attendee. It was like my family and friends didn't want to spend the extra money on a place setting for someone they knew wouldn't be around in the long run.

I decided it was time for a new challenge.

†

When an opportunity came in October 2013 for a position at yet another prestigious federal agency, I immediately prepared my application. The job was competitive, with tens of thousands of applications received each year and a rigorous interview process. On the day of the interview, I had a fever and bronchitis, and I spent the whole day praying I wouldn't cough up a lung in my interviewer's face. I had to stand out among so many candidates, but that was not the way I wanted to achieve it. I survived the eight-hour interview and test in what now seems like a blur. I crashed into bed as soon as I was home, exhausted but smiling. I knew I had done well. God was in control that day.

In January 2014, I received the confirmation letter of employment in the mail. I couldn't have been more excited. With this new job, I saw myself traveling the world using my Arabic language skills. Had I returned to New York, I knew I could have pursued a partner-track position at a private law firm, making more money, maybe even handling high-profile cases. But this was not a job to turn down.

Getting this job, despite all the setbacks I had faced, was such a validation for me. I had just ended yet another relationship and was looking forward to a change. It was the new beginning I had been hoping and praying for. Everything felt right: a new job, remission, a whole new outlook on life. God was rewarding me for returning to Him, time and time again, through my trials. It renewed my faith that I was following the right path.

In February 2014, I hired a realtor and found a condo in Alexandria, Virginia, near the coveted Old Town neighborhood. It was perfect—a one-bedroom in a small community filled with childless, young professionals. And lots of dogs. There was a gym and a pool, and Washington, DC was only a short cab ride away for work or a night on the town. By May, I had closed on the unit and moved in. I was a permanent Virginia resident and finally on my way to "my perfect life." With my new job came new insurance, and with the cancer gone for two years, I no longer thought I needed the fancy insurance I had been paying for. Being treated at a "one-stop shop" clinic where all my providers were under one roof and could share my medical records also appealed to me. When you have cancer, it doesn't just affect one part of your body. You need a range of specialists: oncology, cardiology, pulmonology, gastroenterology, pharmacy. Your entire body becomes a war zone, leaving damaging effects that can last a lifetime.

Most notable of my new in-network doctors was my cardiologist—an optimistic person, which was a quality I really appreciated at the time. On the first visit, he reviewed my medical history, scans, and reports, and concluded I did not need a heart transplant. He thought the previous prognosis six years ago was bogus; it even upset him a little. I'd had none of the characteristic symptoms of heart failure—water retention, kidney problems, or swelling of joints—for more than five years.

He was quite hopeful that if I continued my medications and started a mild cardio regimen, my heart would restore itself.

This doctor believed my ejection fraction could go back up to as much as 60 percent. My resting heart rate, however, was still about 112. It should have been in the seventies. The combination of a high heart rate and a low ejection fraction is like living life in a constant state of fight or flight. I was perpetually out of breath with my heart running in overtime. There was no peace and calm. It was hard to imagine living like this for the next twenty or thirty years, and the prospect deflated my newfound optimism. Even if I survived the cancer, my heart and lungs would still define me as a disabled person. It wasn't a life I wanted. My prayer *take me or heal me* wasn't just a request to be free of the cancer. It was a request to heal *me* in my entirety. I needed to be a whole person.

The rapidness of my heart rate plus a low ejection fraction made my new cardiologist nervous, and every time I went to see him, he urged me to get a defibrillator, which I always politely declined. The following year saw my ejection fraction increase to 45 percent, and he proudly informed me I was out of the danger zone and no longer needed a defibrillator.

But even with all the wins stacking up in my life, something was still missing . . . I needed someone to share it with. I dated two vastly different men around this time. I met Mark on eHarmony. He was a helicopter pilot, tall and attractive, if a little rough around the edges. Not the usual polished professional I dated. Tom, on the other hand, fit the professional image, but lacked the ambition and excitement for life that I have. Both relationships ended within a year, after the revelation that they wanted children and I did not. Or could not, rather.

It was not always a pleasant conversation.

One night after dinner, Tom opened up to me in a way his stoic persona didn't usually allow. "You know," he told me over his third glass of Cab Suav. "I'm forty-five and at my age, I'd sort of given up on getting married." I perked up. Maybe it was the full moon, although most likely it was the wine.

"Until I met you. Since we've started dating, I've started dreaming again." He put down the glass and looked at me shyly. "Marriage. Family. Children. I see it as a possibility now."

The weight of his confession sat on my shoulders, an oppressive cloak. I hated what I was about to say. What I knew I had to say.

"Tom, I can't have children. And I'm not sure I want them at this point. I don't think it's fair with my health history. I may not be around to be a mother to that child."

The light went out of his eyes, and he fell back against his chair. He downed the wine still in his glass, mouth tightening into a thin, hard line. "That dream was short-lived," he snapped.

"Thanks for that."

The bitterness in his voice was harsh and hard to ignore. He resented me for crushing his dream. I thought, *I'm sorry my cancer is an inconvenience to you.* But I didn't say those words out loud. There was no point.

I had enough heartache and disappointments in my own life. I didn't want to be responsible for Tom missing out on something he wanted, and I didn't want to deal with his resentment if we somehow managed to stay together.

A relationship can't survive a confession like that, so we broke up shortly after.

I always told myself I did not want children. I learned at twenty-five I could not have them so, maybe at first, it was something I said to make myself feel better, and I started to believe it over the years. Or maybe God shielded me from the hurt and disappointment of that loss by not putting the instinct or desire in me. I think about that often. Can you grieve something you never had?

I love my niece and nephews; I dote over them as any aunt would. However, the thought of being responsible twenty-four seven for the care of another human is daunting and overwhelming. Perhaps my judgment is biased because of my history now. I have been the person needing care and know the hardship that can put on a family. I've seen the strain on my parents and siblings. Yes, it's different. A child will grow into independence. But they need a strong parent in their lives to raise them to that point.

However, I didn't know if I would live long enough to see a child to maturity. Could I bring them into this world only to leave them too soon? It seemed cruel.

I felt much the same about dating. I don't know if I didn't see Mark and Tom as marriage material, or if I didn't see myself as being available for the long-term commitment marriage required. Again and again, the doctors had put an expiration date on my life: three months, two years, five years. Could I stand before God and my family and make a vow of "until death do us part" when that day hovered large and looming?

So, I made excuses. I dated the wrong men. I sabotaged my own relationships so there wouldn't be the necessity to make any hard choices. Because really wanting something when you knew you couldn't have it hurt too much. Therefore, I rejected the idea before it rejected me.I'd enjoyed the lunches and brunches I'd shared with the men I'd met, getting to know them over football games or dinner and a movie. But it rarely went beyond the initial stages of dating because I did not see my future, any future. I was not giving 100 percent to these relationships because I knew, in my heart, I would not be around for long. Even with Tom and Mark, I was getting stuck around the year mark, and getting over that anniversary hump was always a challenge for me.

I was always waiting for the other shoe to drop.

✝

In January 2016, I joined a new church called DC Metro and became part of a small all-female group that focused on being prosperous in terms of relationships, health, and finances. There were about eight of us at different stages of life, but we all had one thing in common—a desire to gain knowledge in the benefits of biblical teachings to live a more prosperous life. Our conversations revolved around keeping our thoughts and actions centered on the positive and using that, coupled with faith, to attract what we wanted out of life. With "the faith of a mustard seed," we could move mountains.

I loved that group. I practiced my prosperity mantra every day and felt my relationship with God continue to deepen. I also met a new friend, Marie. We instantly became close and she helped me grow my faith, as every sentence out of her mouth either began or ended with, "the Lord willing." She even fasted for my health! For three weeks, from 7 a.m. until 7 p.m., she didn't eat or drink while praying diligently for my healing. A part of me was always in awe of her faith. To this day, I have never fasted. I claim that it's because I am on so many medications, that fasting is not good for me . . . but I wonder if I'm only telling myself that because I don't like feeling hungry. Maybe I will fast someday. But I did have my own experience that increased my faith.

I am an early riser. On one particular Sunday morning, I woke up extra early. Not wanting to fall back asleep, I went to a nearby café to do my daily devotions. That morning, I read a woman's account of how, when she prays to God, He hears her and immediately replies. I felt like she was bragging. I had never experienced that and felt a pang of jealousy. I closed my devotions that morning with a prayer, telling God I didn't feel like he heard me, or more importantly, spoke back.

That morning, at the 9 a.m. service, the pastor stopped in the middle of his sermon and told us a story about how he'd had leukemia when he was fifteen. Completely unrelated to his sermon, it was an abrupt change with no transition, and left the audience looking around with confused faces. He finished his story, recalling how, when he was days away from death in a hospital bed, he was suddenly and inexplicably healed. His cancer never returned. His closing words were, "If you are dealing with cancer, you are going to be healed. You will not die from this. Come see me after church, and I will pray with you." I found him after the service and he prayed for me.

Amazed and unable to shake the experience from my mind as I moved on with my weekend chores, I called Marie, who was still fasting for me.

"Rinad," she said, "I went to the 10:30 sermon, and he didn't bring up that story. I think God heard you and responded to your request."

Looking back, I believe He did hear me, but the answer He would give in the coming months was not the one I had expected . . . or wanted.

Memorial Day weekend in May 2016, I was spending the night at my cousin Rana's house, and a friend had brought all the fixings for ice cream shakes. I might've been the only person on the planet who didn't enjoy ice cream, but somehow, they talked me into trying one. It was the first ice cream shake of my life, and it was delicious— Snickers ice cream blended with chopped nuts, chocolate syrup, and ice. I gulped it down, which was a huge mistake.

I woke up at 2 a.m. and started coughing up blood. Rana heard me and came in to find about half a pint of blood in her bathroom sink. She freaked out worse than me, so to calm her down, I told her I'd had an allergic reaction to the ice cream shake. It wasn't a complete fabrication—I was lactose intolerant.

I called my primary care provider first thing in the morning, who ordered an X-ray and told me to come in immediately. I was running late for work and told her I would come in later. Completely stupefied by my nonchalance, Rana rearranged her schedule and dragged me to the appointment. The X-ray was enough for my doctor to refer me to a pulmonologist, who discovered my right lung had completely collapsed again, due to the presence of an enormous mass. She ordered a biopsy, which came back negative for lung cancer. I was diagnosed with a severe case of pulmonary fibrosis and needed to get on the lung transplant list immediately. I reminded her I was only four years into my required five years of cancer remission and asked if I could have the mass removed instead. She advised against removal due to the size of the mass and damage already done to the lungs from the talc, and recommended I get a PET scan to confirm I was still in remission in order to get a spot on the list. I got the scan.

My life shattered again.

It showed that the Hodgkin's had returned. I went into shock. Something inside me shut down. I couldn't believe it. I didn't believe it. I was in remission. This was supposed to be behind me. I rejected the offers to have the lymph nodes around the lung biopsied to confirm the diagnosis. I couldn't fathom that I actually had cancer again.

Then I got a call from my uncle and he was completely shaken. A physician himself, he'd been with me from the beginning, through every diagnosis and treatment, and the changes in jobs and insurance and doctors. He often got the information about my prognosis before I did because doctors are more likely to talk to other doctors.

Nothing rattles my uncle, but he had called the pulmonologist himself to get the full story, and painted a pretty grim picture of what would happen if I didn't have the biopsy. It was not just my lung at risk, but my spleen and stomach as well. At his insistence, I got the additional biopsy and, lo and behold, the diagnosis was confirmed. At that moment, if the Earth had crumbled beneath my feet, I might not have noticed it.

Back in 2012, when I was pronounced in remission, I threw a Blessings Party to thank God, my family, and my friends for their love and support during my—at that time—nine-year ordeal. It was a very elaborate and fancy event. I rented out a restaurant venue and hosted a four-course sit down dinner. I wore a long, gold-sequined gown. The men wore suits and ties, and the ladies were in cocktail dresses. There was an open bar and even a champagne toast.

It was in every way the wedding reception I believed I should have had by then and might never get. But mostly I was so thankful to God for bringing me through.

When I found out I was sick again, I felt God had betrayed me. We'd had a deal. I went through hell for nine years and, for the most part, kept my faith. I actually told God He owed me $2,000 for the money I spent on the Blessings Party—the party I threw to honor Him! How dare He put me in this position again! Hadn't I already learned whatever cosmic lesson He was trying to teach me?

Why me? I started asking again.

This was not the usual "Why me?" question one asks when illness falls on them, but "Why me?" as in "Why am I still alive?" Why does God keep pushing me to the brink of death only to catapult me back? Why are people dying from this disease or other tragedies, but I am still around year after year circling the same mountain? Is it survivor's guilt? Should I feel guilty I am still here?

The answer, apparently, was a resounding "no."

CHAPTER 27

Google, My Doctor's Savior

Again, I found myself at a familiar crossroads: which treatment to choose to fight the cancer and hopefully not die.

This time, I had three options. The first was to take the same drug I had taken back in 2012 that had put me in remission, Brentuximab. Since it had been four years since last taking this drug, I was a viable candidate to do it again. The second was immunotherapy, which had just been approved for treating Hodgkin's a few months prior. And third was a Phase I experimental drug study, which at that time had "delivered good results in mice with limited side effects." Ever the diligent problem-solver, I started gathering as much information as I could on each of the options, then met with Dr. T, the head of the lymphoma department, to discuss which path I should take. His response left me absolutely floored.

After reviewing my files, he put my folder aside. "I can't advise you on what to do."

I waited for the "but," followed by some kind advice. None came. After recovering from my stunned silence, I asked him, "What would you say to your daughter if she was in the same position?"

His face was as blank as a new piece of paper. "I don't have kids."

"Your niece, then?" Hoping for something, anything resembling guidance.

"I'm an only child."

So, that's who I was dealing with.

When I asked him about the immunotherapy option, that it looked promising and I wanted more details, he said he didn't know. He then turned to his monitor and searched for the information on Google. When I asked about the dosage being used in the study, he had to look that up as well. Did he think I was looking for a study buddy?

But I learned something valuable from this interaction: There is a thing in the medical industry called *first-line oncologists*, physicians who are just there to provide rudimentary information and then refer you onto someone worth their salt. He was one of them.

The one useful thing he did tell me was that, since I had relapsed with the Brentuximab, I would never be cured unless I got a bone marrow transplant. When I reminded him that every other doctor had told me my heart and lungs were not strong enough for a transplant, he doubled back into his protective shell of no further advice. The only good that came out of this conversation was the introduction to the most competent and intelligent doctor I have ever crossed paths with, Dr. Spira.

My appointment with this doctor in Virginia where the Phase I trial was being conducted was a completely different experience. It was quite the opposite, in fact. Dr. Spira took time to listen to my story, read all my reports, and view all my scans and past treatments.

"The trial is new," he advised. "And I'm reluctant to have you join since we don't yet know the effect on humans. You still have other viable options, so I would recommend you wait. Phase I studies are more suited to patients who have exhausted all other treatment options."

It was a refreshing change. With his easy yet confident personality, he likely could have persuaded me to join and help fill the required seats in his trial. But he didn't, instead putting my best interests first, the way every doctor should.

Between the Brentuximab or immunotherapy, he felt both were viable. But since I had gone into remission with Brentuximab before, that might be the better choice. If it put me in remission again, it could give the trial enough time to conclude, and by then, it might be the cure I needed. He was also the first physician who refused to give me a prognosis on my life. He refused to say how long he thought I had to live, stating that every person reacts differently to diseases and their treatments. This was my first good experience with an oncologist. It was so good that I switched insurance, again, to make him my primary oncologist.

I was still feeling a little uneasy about which avenue to take, so I reached out to a couple of friends I had known since my first year in pre-med at George Washington back in 1997. Not only had they gotten married, but both went on to become doctors. They had tracked my progress for years and were always happy to be sounding boards for me.

They referred me to an oncologist friend of theirs for another opinion. At this point, I was using every tool in my belt.

This new doctor agreed that either Brentuximab or immunotherapy would be the best option and leaned more toward Brentuximab because it had put me in remission before and could do it again. He cautioned, though, that I would likely relapse again, and my only cure would be a bone marrow transplant if my heart and lungs were strong enough for it.

I couldn't make a decision. In some ways, I wanted God to take this decision out of my hands. In the past, I'd jumped when doctors told me to. I repeatedly allowed myself to be rushed into choosing a treatment, and too often, I regretted the decision. Now, I was doing research to make a fully informed decision, but in truth, the way I chose to cope with the uncertainty was to ignore it. Honestly, I was waiting for peace to come over either decision, and it never happened.

My uncertainty here was mirrored in my personal life as well. I'd begun dating Jason, a Christian man I'd met through OKCupid. Everything was going great for the first two months, but when I got the cancer diagnosis, he changed in an instant.

Jason, for all his claims of faith, didn't show a very Christian attitude. He was constantly late or standing me up for planned nights out. And he would give a lame excuse or no excuse at all. It was like he was testing me, daring me to break up with him, since he didn't have the guts to do it himself.

After a month of going back and forth about which treatment option I should pursue, I decided I needed a vacation to clear my head and make a sound decision. I had a friend who lived in Santa Barbara and my sister also had a friend whose father was an oncologist and lived an hour from Santa Barbara. I organized a visit in June 2016, packed my bag, and jumped on a plane to hopefully find the peace I needed to make a decision.

Meeting with the oncologist in California would prove highly informative. I learned that one of the side effects from the immunotherapy is pneumonitis, a lung disease caused by inflammation or irritation in the lungs. This doctor said it ordinarily happens in only a small number of patients, but since I already had lung disease, my chances increased from nil to 90 percent. With pneumonitis, I would not be able to breathe without assistance, and it would not go away until the treatment was finished. He didn't believe I would be able to finish the regimen without being a prisoner of the hospital relying on breathing machines. To him, I was too young to chance such severe complications for so little hope of reward, since a cure was not in my cards without the bone marrow transplant.

I was still uncertain on a direction, so after I left his office, I called another uncle, who was a pharmacist, and asked him to run the drugs for the three options through his system at work to see what the side effects of each were. He faxed me reports on each, and we went over them together.

Reading the material, I saw everything from neuropathy to autoimmune disorders, including arthritis, colitis, pneumonitis, or any other "-itis" where the body begins attacking itself. Even though the pneumonitis is reversible, I did not want to risk further damage to my lungs. It was beginning to feel like I was playing a dangerous game of body-part roulette. And the last option, the Phase I drug study, was a complete unknown.

My uncle agreed with Dr. Spira, that I should use one of the other two options to get to remission again; then hopefully, there would be new treatments besides a bone marrow transplant if I relapsed again. Or, at the very least, the drug trial would gain notoriety and we would be able to see its side effects and efficacy on actual humans.

The trip to California proved successful, and though there were still obvious risks, I decided I would start taking Brentuximab. I called my doctor and told him to start the insurance authorization process. He was hesitant, reminding me that this was not a full cure, that a bone marrow transplant was the only hope for a cure, and because of that, I may not get insurance approval for any other treatment. The Brentuximab had been tried before to no avail, and other options were available that could work better. He requested I visit a former colleague at the very same prestigious hospital where I had tried to get an appointment years prior, but was rejected. He hoped the doctors there could talk some sense into me about the transplant. Finally! I'd been trying to see a doctor at this facility for ages.

I agreed to go, but for my own reason—to get him to write a note stating my heart and lungs were too weak for a bone marrow transplant and that starting Brentuximab was my only viable option. I would show this letter to the insurance company to get the approval I needed to start Brentuximab treatments ASAP.

This doctor, although clearly very bright, spun in like the Tasmanian Devil, spoke really fast, then was out the door again before I could even blink. It was a whirlwind of an appointment, and gave me no new information, except that the MVP treatment I had taken eleven years earlier—the one that was not FDA-approved for Hodgkin's Lymphoma— had been considered ahead of its time. My doctor (Dr. W from the Bronx) was a genius for prescribing it to me. A lot of good that did me to know, considering I still had cancer and a lot of terrible, irreversible side effects from that awful cocktail.

One other thing he said was that my heart and lungs were not too weak. In fact, if I was breathing on my own, then I could handle the transplant. He had patients in far worse conditions than me, ones having to be wheeled in for appointments because their pulmonary or cardiac capabilities were so diminished, who survived the transplant procedure. I chose to ignore him because I knew in my gut the transplant was not the way to go.

Also, I read reports on patients developing graft-versus-host disease, a condition that occurs when donor bone marrow or stem cells attack the recipient cells. It occurs in as many as four out of five transplant recipients, causing a range of medical problems. In certain cases, this could be more painful than the chemo that is administered before the transplant to completely obliterate the body's immune system. I was prone to every imaginable, and sometimes unimaginable, side effect from every treatment, drug, or procedure, so I did not want to put my body through that.

After I declined for the third time, he irately said I would be dead in three months if I did not take the bone marrow transplant option. I thanked him for his time and he tornadoed out the door as dramatically as he'd spun in.

I returned to Dr. T and informed him, resolutely, that I was not getting a bone marrow transplant and that Dr. Spira agreed it was a good decision to do the Brentuximab. If insurance decided not to pay for it, I would wait until January when my new insurance kicked in and try again. He requested approval, and I received it immediately. I started treatment the following week.

This also seemed to shake loose the uncertainty I had over Jason. While struggling with the decision over which treatment to select, I realized my weakened heart and one working lung made me physically less than a whole person. But I still deserved to be treated like a whole person. Jason didn't seem capable of doing that, so I called it quits.

My time for settling was over—on men and doctors.

CHAPTER 28

A Hairy Situation

My never-ending battle with cancer was holding center stage in my life yet again, but this time I had reason to hope. I had been down the road of Brentuximab before and had found remission. And since my body had tolerated it so well the first time, I thought treatment would be a relative walk in the park.

Why I continually set myself up for disappointment like that, I don't think I'll ever know.

During my first treatment, I started itching and developed a rash all over my body. The nurses gave me Benadryl, which only made the reaction worse. I got cold and clammy and my heart started beating erratically. I tried to scream, but nothing came out. I couldn't breathe. I gasped for air and flailed my arms. Aunt Ellen was with me, and the last thing I remember seeing was the look of horror on her face as the world went dark.

Something flickered in me in those last moments of consciousness: I wanted to survive. I'd fought too long and too hard to get to this point in life. Even if I'd had my doubts, in the end I'd always chosen to keep fighting. I was worth fighting for. I wanted to wake up and continue to fight this illness—to continue to live my life with purpose. The nurses revived me, and that's what I did.

Two hours later, we slowly started the drip again. Six hours later, I had completed the entire course. The doctor explained that I'd had an anaphylactic reaction because my body must have built antibodies against the carrier that transported the chemo when I first took the Brentuximab back in 2011, so it was now recognizing and rejecting it. He assured me the chemo inside would be safely transported to the infected lymph nodes. Trusting the doctor's statement, I felt a little better about the first treatment. I was a little queasy, like you might feel after a long night of tequila shots. But on the whole, I was confident.

After five days, I started losing my hair. It was time to shop for a wig again. This was not a part of my plan, especially since I did not lose my hair the first time I took Brentuximab. In fact, I was promised that hair loss was not a side effect. This mystified both Dr. T and Dr. Spira because no patient up until that point had ever reported hair loss while on Brentuximab. I was a medical marvel yet again, and not the good kind!

To distract myself before treatments began, I had joined Bumble, a dating app, and had started seeing William. We had only gone on a few dates, but how was I supposed to explain the journey to baldness? The first date we had, before my hair started falling out, was a four-hour marathon date. Four hours is a long time to notice the physical characteristics of a person, and specifically whether or not she is bald. Something like that would stand out.

The second date happened while my hair was clumping out. I was able to part it in a way that hid the bald spots, but I still had to cut my hair shorter because it looked too wispy at the length it was. By the third date, I was completely bald, and I needed to wear a wig. More importantly, I needed a convincing story that explained why, on three separate dates in a two-week timeframe, I had three distinct haircuts.

I found myself having yet another breakdown tied around my hair loss. I pretended to be a regular thirty-something woman living a normal life, but I was anything but a normal thirty-something.

Dating was my release, my way to get away, and if I was no longer able to date casually, what outlet did I have? In the end, I told William I had always wanted short hair, but was afraid to cut it all at once. I was doing it in phases to make sure it was what I wanted. Did that make me commitment-phobic? Was I just another squirrely woman from an internet dating site obscuring her looks? I wore my wig, continued to date him, and hoped he would buy the story. I realize now I probably spent way more time thinking about my hair than he did.

The most traumatizing thing about losing my hair was that, when I had hair, I could act like I didn't have cancer. It was as if I were Samson and my identity, and emotional strength, were found in my hair. Once it was lost, I would lose all my superpowers and the world would know. They would know my weakness. They would know I was sick. They would know I was a fraud.

✝

It was a hard time in my life since I was out on medical leave and trying to manage having neither work nor studies to consume my thoughts for the first time since I was four years old. As I continued treatment, my condition steadily worsened. After my third treatment, I developed a high fever and shortness of breath. My temperature spiked to 102°F, and since it was Friday night, and my insurance required pre-approval before admittance to an actual hospital—which I could not receive until Monday morning—I had to settle for an urgent care facility.

When I was checked in to my room, I met with the doctor and very matter-of-factly gave him my symptoms and told him I was certain I had pneumonia. I'd experienced the same symptoms a dozen times in the past. I knew what I was talking about. He listened to my lungs and said they were clear and the X-ray showed I did not have pneumonia. He confirmed I had a fever and was neutropenic, but was adamant I did not have pneumonia. He listened several times, at my insistence, since I could feel the wheezing and crackling in my chest, but he would not change his mind. I grew agitated. I knew these symptoms and knew I had pneumonia. I asked to be seen by another doctor.

Another one came, but agreed with the original doctor. She did not hear any wheezing. She looked at the X-ray and saw no signs of pneumonia. She gave me an IV antibiotic for the neutropenia and left. The first doctor returned and said my shortness of breath could be an anxiety attack and gave me something to treat anxiety, even though I told him I was not crazy. I insisted I needed a CT scan to confirm pneumonia. He proceeded to order a CT scan, but with an angiogram to see if there was a blood clot, which made absolutely no sense, given I had pneumonia. Then he left, and I never saw him again.

As soon as the morning rolled around, I came to learn I did, in fact, have pneumonia, but that doctor did not come in and admit to his misdiagnosis. I sat in a cold room all night thinking I was going crazy. This happened so often that I didn't even react anymore; it was like I'd come to expect this. This is terribly sad, seeing as how we live in the strongest economy in the world with world-class medical facilities filled with state of the art equipment, but the bedside manner is lacking.

I was discharged at 10 a.m. on Saturday after another round of IV antibiotics, though I still had a fever. And pneumonia. And was still neutropenic. I was told my PCP would contact me on Monday to see how I was doing.

The urgent care doctor told me to track my fever and return to the urgent care facility if my fever persisted. My fever persisted for five days, but I did not return to that clinic. I think, at the time, I believed I was safer at home, even though there were some nights I didn't think I would make it through. Over the next few days, before the fever broke, I was unable to walk from the toilet to my bed without collapsing and hyperventilating.

The reality was I should never have been discharged from a doctor's care until the fever had completely subsided. Furthermore, once my PCP heard that the fever lingered many days, she said I should have been admitted to the cancer wing of a real hospital. But neither of those things happened, and I believe it was only the grace of God that saved me.

My aunt called my parents from urgent care to let them know I had pneumonia, and immediately, my dad offered to come and stay with me. I declined, but he came anyway, and I'm so glad he did. There are times when a girl just needs her father, whether she's six or thirty-six.

On the evening after I had been released, he called from Union Station. He was getting in a cab and on his way to visit me. When he called again to tell me he was nearly there, I went outside and waited for him, but he didn't arrive. I called him back, and he told me he had passed through the gate and was outside of my building complex.

Now, my condo complex is very large and includes eight different buildings. I did not have the energy to walk around the entire complex, so I kept calling and finally told him to ask the next random passerby for help. He put a gentleman on the phone, and it turns out, my dad had written the wrong number down; he was standing in front of 3305 and I was in 3315. This kind man walked him to my doorstep.

My dad spent two weeks with me. He cooked fresh soups and Jordanian dishes. He went grocery shopping and cleaned my place. He was truly the rock I needed so I could focus on my healing. But most of all, he kept me company while also giving me the space a sick person needs to heal.

While my father was staying with me, a gentleman I met on Bumble contacted me. Once we got through the initial formalities, we began chatting and talking about where we lived. I gave him a general location, not yet sure I wanted to pursue an in-person meetup. To my surprise, he said he lived nearby. When I named the street, he said he lived there as well and gave me the name of my complex. I asked which building, and he said 3305. Completely blown away, I responded with 3315. He then proceeded to tell me that a few days prior, he had helped a nice, older man find 3315. He was the guy who helped my dad get to me. I thanked him profusely for helping my dad, telling him he had really saved the day for us that afternoon.

He asked me out on a date for that weekend, but I still had pneumonia and couldn't meet anyone yet. By the time I was better, he was nowhere to be found.

I often wondered whether he had been sent for the sole purpose of getting my father to my building, kind of my own guardian angel. Maybe our connection through the dating app was just my opportunity to say thank you to this kind person for helping a stranger in need. This was yet another confirmation that God was watching over me, putting the right people in my life when they were needed. I didn't always know the purpose they would serve, but I knew there was a reason we crossed paths. There is a truth to the mysteries of God, and we just have to trust in it.

At one point, while my dad was staying with me, my fever spiked again, but I refused to tell him. I knew in my heart that if I went back to that urgent care facility, I would die anyway, and I had a better chance of staying alive if I remained at home. With my father in the next room, I had a sense of peace that if I died, I would not die alone. It gave me the serenity I needed to rest and heal.

As you already know, I did not die that night, or in the nights to follow. After two weeks of good food and healthy living, my Baba nursed me back to health. The fever subsided and I was out of the danger zone. I completed one final treatment. Three weeks later, a scan showed that the masses were unchanged, and I was in remission.

But there was a caveat, and the doctors made this abundantly clear. The treatment I had just finished was only a temporary fix. The cancer would return within two to five years. At that time, if a new cure had not presented itself, a bone marrow transplant would be my only option. But I couldn't be bothered with such warnings. I was in remission again.

God had a plan for me, again, and all my hard work was not going to go to waste.

Life #8

CHAPTER 29

Kicking the Bucket List

Shortly after my dad nursed me back to health, I was officially in remission once again, my umpteenth trip around the mountain. It was hard to get excited, as my attitude was very much a *been there, done that* sort of thing. In some ways this relapse had been harder to deal with, having broken my four-year streak. The magical fifth year, the finish line when I could start planning for the heart and lung transplant, had been within my grasp. Hope had once again seduced me like the temptress it was—promising, luring me in, almost within my grasp—and had been snatched away in the final hours.

My family and I decided to take a vacation in December 2016. A variety of reasons were behind the trip, but my sinking mood and precarious health surely topped the list. The three-week-long, epic vacation began with a visit to my younger brother in Abu Dhabi. Danny, the only one of us who was American-born, had gone to the United Arab Emirates as a real estate consultant.

Next was Jordan, where we did all the touristy stuff: posh hotels, the Dead Sea, the River Jordan, and the Holy Sites. I got to see the home where my mom and aunt were raised; the same house near where I had been born on the kitchen floor.

My thoughts lingered on my mother and the journey that had brought her from a small town in Jordan to the East Coast of the United States. She was one in a family of nine. At school, her friends called her Jidda, or "grandmother" in Arabic. She was not only incredibly caring and loving, giving her a maternal energy, but she possessed wisdom and intuition beyond her years.

She was also a rule breaker, or at least a rule bender, which is where I'm sure I get it from. When she left high school, she attended the Beirut Arab University's Amman satellite campus, which gave her the opportunity to travel to Beirut, Lebanon, every semester to complete her practicums. She channeled all of that care, love, and wisdom into studying to become a teacher. During the summers, she was a teacher's aide, putting into practice what she had learned.

She'd gone against the norms for young girls in her day—putting marriage on hold, leaving home to study. Later, when it would have been easy to give in to the dictates of culture and pressure from family, she fought to let my sister and I do the same if that was what we wanted.

It takes an incredible amount of strength and courage to stand against expectations. *Go with the flow. Don't rock the boat.* All are sayings meant to keep the peace. Mom wasn't exactly a peacekeeper, preferring to do the things she knew were best for her family.

We also visited my dad's family home. During high school, Air Force recruiters came to his high school and saw in him what his parents knew all along—he was a mature young man capable of anything. He dropped out of high school early to join the Royal Jordanian Air Force. In doing so, he turned himself from a high school boy into a good-looking, self-made young man who was ready to settle down.

My parents met while my father's family was visiting my mother's family to explore an engagement between her brother and his sister. It was a surprise reunion, since my mother hadn't laid eyes on my father since grade school years prior. But they started talking and realized they had a lot in common, besides both being single Christians and of a suitable age to marry.

The four of them settled on a double wedding, inviting the entire town to celebrate the unions. My father continued working for the Air Force and my mother began building the foundation of our little family. A year later, my oldest brother, Tariq, was born. My mother had taken a break from college for marriage and pregnancy, and after she gave birth, she finished her degree.

I think about how difficult it must have been as a mother and a student at just twenty years old. A few years after graduating, she became pregnant with my sister, Loren. It's hard for me to envision the juggling act she must have gone through at such a young age. At twenty—focused on my studies, friends, boys—I was still finding myself. I cannot imagine trying to figure out who I should be while bringing new people into this world. Perhaps you can see why my mother is so inspiring to me.

In my own way, I liked to think I was honoring their legacy—built decades ago in a land sometimes torn apart by religious persecution and political differences—with my latest decisions in terms of treating the cancer. While I'd gotten my persistence and fearlessness from my mother, my father had gifted me with the ability to figure things out along the way, learning not to make the same mistakes again.

I don't think I had failed them with my earlier choices. I was doing my best to survive, to make my way through this journey on faith and instinct. My strength was born from two people who made strong choices against all odds. I could do no less.

After Jordan, we went to Dubai to visit my older brother and his family. My sister joined us from New York, and we spent Christmas on the beach in 85°F weather. It was a day to remember.

This trip was important to me. When you have a disease like cancer, you look at things and wonder if this will be the last time . . . the last Christmas, the last visit home, the last sunset. I'd accepted the eventuality of my early death. I did not know when or if I would have another opportunity to visit my homeland with my parents. Again, I did not know how long I or they would be around. I relished this time to see and visit places that had shaped my parents into the incredible people they are.

CHAPTER 30

Mr. Make-A-Wish Come True

Family was not the only thing on my mind while I was away. After the unsuccessful dating attempts with Jason, Tom, and Mark, I was a little gun shy about going back to the usual online sites. As my father had taught me, I didn't want to keep repeating the same mistakes. But like my mother, I wasn't giving up. Meeting the right person was more important than ever. Given the most recent events with my disease and treatments, I felt the ticking clock present more than ever.

I thought about an article I had read on dating with intention, as well as how to prepare myself to be the person I wanted my future partner to meet. My faith was strong. I was independent in spite of my health. I was successful. I gave back through my volunteer work with Christian Legal Aid and Make-A-Wish Foundation. I was trying to be less selfish.

I tried to zero in on those qualities that really mattered to me in my future spouse. I thought back to the list I'd made so many years ago when thinking of the perfect man for me. I wanted someone kind, generous, successful, faithful.

Before my family vacation, I had met a guy named Bertrand on Bumble. He was attractive, and we had a lot in common politically. Our first date was the night after the most contentious and controversial presidential election in US history, and we spent the whole dinner talking about the one thing you shouldn't discuss on dates—politics.

I liked him. He was forty-six, good-looking, and successful. Although it was a fantastic date, when we parted ways, I figured I would never see him again. He had never married, and I assumed it was a choice he'd made consciously, something he was not interested in. I wrote him off as a playboy bachelor since I was looking for the opposite end of the spectrum. I didn't think our paths would cross again. I had little time to waste on a relationship that was not going to end with a ring on my finger.

I was nursing pneumonia at the time, so I was a bit aloof on the first date. Again, it wasn't that I didn't like him; I thought we had different goals. I had spent years investing time in relationships for the short-term to lull the loneliness, while losing sight of my long-term desire to get married. I wasn't about to do that again. And instinct was telling me to get out early if this relationship seemed like it would go nowhere.

Three weeks later, when I was well enough to go out again, Bertrand and I met for a second date over brunch. Always the perfectionist, I needed to get all the facts for my decision before I wrote him off as the Romeo I'd pegged him to be.

I mentioned my volunteer work with the Make-A-Wish Foundation, and explained that volunteering there was important to me on so many levels. Besides the obvious—getting to help sick children and families in need—it was also helping me heal. As a survivor of cancer, and as someone trying daily to be a good Christian, I was left with the question: Can you be a good person while fighting to save your own life? Volunteering with Make-A-Wish was my way of proving it was possible—a way to be less self-involved when stuck with such a selfish disease.

I told him how Make-A-Wish had run out of funding and one of my Wish Kids had to have a trip postponed. To my surprise, Bertrand immediately offered to send the family a check to cover the expenses.

I was so surprised by the words uttered by my date that I nearly fell off my chair, spewing the croquette out of my mouth. "You want to do what?"

Bertrand handed me a napkin without batting an eye. "I want to donate to your Make-A-Wish family. It's clearly important to you, so it's important to me. And I am in a position to help. Tell me how much is needed and where to send it, and I'll cut a check."

Something clicked in me in that moment. I remembered my belief that God puts the right people in my life at the right time. Was Bertrand one of those people? Was he here to help me get my Wish Kid the planned trip? Or was there something more? I found myself hoping for the latter. Was I looking at the kind and generous man I had been searching for and, quite honestly, not expecting to find?

This was the first time I am glad to say I did not trust my instinct to run like I wanted to when I first met him. He was on my mind the whole time I was away in Dubai.

When we met for the first time, I had been almost completely bald and in a wig. But there was no way I was telling him my complete story. I didn't want to scare him off. Did I look like someone with cancer? Could he tell? Keeping a secret is a heavy burden; it gains weight with the keeping. I've learned that sharing it shares the burden. I'd not had many people to share this journey with over the years, and when I did share, the heavy lifting was spread out.

Despite my fixation on the what-ifs, based on my experiences telling previous dates of my situation, this felt different. When I thought of telling Bertrand, an unusual lightness would fill me.

Before I needed to decide, I left on my family vacation, where I continued to wonder how Bertrand would respond if I told him this secret. When I returned to the States, we made plans to meet up, and I can honestly say it was the best New Year's Eve I have ever had. He knew how to make me laugh. With little effort, he could draw me into deep philosophical conversations about the state of the world or the best sushi in New York. I wanted to see more of Bertrand, but the insecurities surrounding my health issues were kicking in full-time.

Looking back, however, it was easy to see Bertrand was not the kind of man to be culled out of my life by something like cancer. He was humble and generous, a truly good person, more interested in what was inside than outside. I wanted him to see that in me as well. Rather than worrying about my hair, I was worried about whom he saw when he looked at me. Was I kind and generous? Was I faithful? You know you're with the right person when you want to be a better person for them.

The big question filling my mind, however, was, *Could he see himself building a future with me, even if that future was limited?*

About three months in, at a wine tasting event one night, we had our first serious conversation about the future. It felt a little like dropping a bomb, then waiting around while it ticked away by your toes.

"Do you want kids?" I asked him, not quite meeting his gaze, but watching his body language from under my lashes.

I think he was nervous because he started talking in a roundabout way. He scratched at the tablecloth and picked at his napkin. "That's a big question. I can't say I haven't thought about it. Men have it easy. They can have kids until their seventies—"

I knew what he was getting at, so I interrupted him. "It's okay; I don't want kids either."

His sigh of relief was audible. But the conversation was just getting started. I needed to be straight with him on what I wanted out of a relationship, and if we didn't want the same things, I knew tonight would be our last date. It hurt more than I wanted to admit when I thought about not seeing him again.

I dropped the m-bomb. I sat up straight in my chair and told him, "I want to get married someday. That is the expectation I have going into any relationship. I'm looking for a partner for life, not just someone to date. If you don't see yourself getting married, then we should end things."

And just like his relief earlier had been instantaneous, his delight matched it. "I would definitely like to find the right person and get married as well."

He went on to explain how he'd been searching all along for that special someone to share his life. He was successful both professionally and personally. He had family and friends, and adored his nieces and nephews. But as time had passed and he hadn't gotten married, he'd slowly accepted it wouldn't happen for him.

"I was okay with that," he said, again not quite meeting my eyes, "until I met you."

In that moment, I knew Bertrand was different from all the other men I'd dated. I knew he was the one for me. When Tom had told me the same thing—he hadn't thought of getting married or starting a family until he'd met me—I was annoyed he was burdening me with his feelings. With Bertrand, I wanted to take away all his past hurts and disappointments.

I could feel my fingers closing in on that elusive temptation of hope dangling so close this time. My nerves really kicked in. It was confession time. What would happen next was going to seal the deal.

I couldn't let the relationship continue without him knowing about my health problems. I'd thought about this a lot over the course of our courtship. In the past, I'd kept my health a secret, and it was like having a third person in the relationship—something that had to be managed and scheduled around, and kept as a dirty little secret. If this was going to work with Bertrand, I had to be honest with him.

I told him a summarized version of my history with cancer. "The last round of treatment caused my hair to fall out." I touched the ends of *my* hair. "This is a wig."

He didn't flinch. I smiled tentatively.

I mentioned my heart and lung issues, and my physical limitations in sparse detail. I didn't want to overwhelm him all at once. "In case you wanted to be with a sporty, active girl, I won't be climbing Mt. Fuji or biking the 100-mile Scary Poodle if that's your thing."

There was no fear in his eyes. "It's not. I can think of plenty of things to do for date nights in DC."

Then I dropped the next bomb. "I'm in remission, but it's not a cure. The doctors think I'll likely relapse in two to five years."

That's when I saw the first glimpse of change in his countenance. It wasn't a look of disgust, or doubt, or a discomfort that spoke of wanting to end the date. It was compassion.

"Doctors don't know everything. And even if it does come back," he reached across the table, grabbing my hand, "they are making medical advances every day."

A broken me wasn't a deal breaker for him.

As hope finally felt firmly in my grasp, I think my heart melted into my chair. I later learned he confided to a friend that he would rather be with me, knowing I might not be around long, than with another girl who had no health problems and was certain to live longer. After forty-six years, he could not see himself with anyone else.

I was right. God had put Bertrand in my life for a reason. That lighter feeling I described? I knew that was God telling me Bertrand wouldn't just share in the knowledge of my disease, but he would help me fight it every step of the way and carry me when needed. I no longer had to do this alone.

I did continue to wear my wig around him until my hair was long enough to rock a natural hairdo eight months later. Some insecurities die hard.

The physical limitations I had glossed over during our wine tasting date came to the forefront during one of our dates to Great Falls on the Billy Goat trail. He'd described it as a four-mile *flat* hike. "More like a walk," he assured me. Determined to at least try, I agreed to the outing and off we went. After three hours, we'd only reached the two-mile marker.

I looked at him angrily. "You said it was flat!"

"It is flat." He was perplexed, I could tell, and was trying to stay calm in the face of my anger and frustration. He was probably also a little scared. What would happen if I couldn't make it back? Visions of search-and-rescue swooping in must have filled his head at that moment; they certainly were filling mine. This was not how I wanted the date to go.

"Climbing rocks uphill is not flat!" I slapped my hand against the boulder on which I'd collapsed. "I only have one functional lung, so climbing stairs or hills is nearly impossible for me."

That was the last time we went hiking, and the first time he got a full glimpse of my physical limitations.

When we finally made it back to the car, we sat silently for a minute, each of us lost in thought. Finally, he said, "I don't mind the things you can't do, but I won't assume. You have to tell me."

And he was right. I needed to be honest with him. I'd been worried about running him off with the truth, but now it seemed I could run him off by withholding the truth.

We continued to see each other periodically over the next several months. Unlike the other men I had dated, he was slow and steady. I actually hated it. *Maybe he isn't interested*, I would tell myself. Though I wasn't used to a slow pace, I liked that he did not put any pressure on me, especially since I had health issues. It gave me the room to really think about what I wanted. Did I really want to be married? Were kids really out of the question, or was it something I told myself because I had been infertile since I was twenty-five, thanks to the MVP cocktail? Possibilities started emerging. Dare I say it . . . hope?

Around that time, I developed a new symptom. Large amounts of mucus would build up in my throat so that I could barely complete a sentence without sounding froggy. A pulmonary test and a few blood tests revealed I had high levels of immunoglobulins, which indicated an allergic reaction to something.

At least that's what the pulmonologist thought.

This prompted more blood tests, which pointed to a severe allergy to mold. She believed mold spores were stuck in my lungs, causing the allergic reaction. She recommended I complete an antifungal regimen, but warned it would be very harsh on my body. Before starting the regimen, I saw an allergy specialist who ran forty-eight environmental allergy tests and fifty-two food allergy tests—that's one hundred needle pricks on my arms, back, and stomach. And after all that, the conclusion was that I had no allergies, not even to mold. The allergy testing further concluded I had no mold in my lungs. The antifungal regimen was not necessary.

Over the next six weeks, I was on a whirlwind tour of different specialists, which included a painful and unnecessary endoscopy. This all resulted in me being diagnosed with acid reflux and a sinus infection. But after two months of antibiotics and antacids, the mucus had not resolved. By August 2017, I was having a hard time breathing and had developed a slight fever. I went back to the pulmonologist and told her I thought I had pneumonia and asked for an X-ray. She listened to my lungs and told me they sounded completely clear. It was not pneumonia, she insisted.

Oh boy, I thought, remembering that horrific night in urgent care. *Not this again.*

I told her my history, but she didn't want me to have to pay for an X-ray I didn't need. She explained that sometimes, with a bad sinus infection, a patient will need several rounds of antibiotics, sometimes taken with steroids to allow the antibiotics to work better. During this two-month period, she diagnosed me with three sinus infections. I was on non-stop antibiotics, each course more aggressive than the one before.

I was going to Costa Rica with Bertrand that weekend and asked her one last time for an X-ray. There was a machine sitting *right there* in her office. She wouldn't budge. She sent me abroad while I had a fever, armed with another round of antibiotics and ten days' worth of steroids. With my extensive history of cancer in my lungs I still find it odd she did not suspect it was lymphoma. She heard hoofbeats and thought zebra.

Even with these issues, I had an amazing time with Bertrand on vacation. The steroids allowed my breathing to clear up, and my fever went away, so we filled our days with the incredible beaches, waterfalls, and hot springs Costa Rica is famous for, as well as plenty of time by the pool. At night, we danced and sat beneath the stars, talking about nothing and everything. In all the ways that counted, we were just like any other couple. I began to get hopeful it was just a sinus infection after all, but when I returned, and the ten-day course of steroids was over, the shortness of breath returned.

I went to see my cardiologist to learn if the shortness of breath could be heart related. He also declared my lungs to be clear and concluded my breathing issue was probably a bad infection, as my heart was fine and not causing fluid to build up. Ironically, he is married to my pulmonologist so part of me thinks he had to agree with her diagnosis. Then, he commented on my high pulse. I told him my resting heart rate had been about 110 to 112 beats per minute since 2010. He was alarmed. He told me about a great medicine that would slow my heart rate down and wanted me to start it. I was shocked. In seven years, not a single one of my doctors offered me this solution.

Grateful at this new discovery, I left the cardiologist's clinic with a new medication treating an old issue, but no answers as to the cause of my shortness of breath. I called my pulmonologist several times during this period to ask for more steroids, which had been the only thing to help, and she didn't call me back. I will never understand this trait in people, especially doctors. Lawyers *love* to call people back. It starts the clock ticking, and since we bill every six minutes, the longer the call, the better. I believe if doctors were paid by the hour, they would be more responsive with patients.

I waited for a couple of weeks, hoping the new cardiac medicine would trigger the shortness of breath to subside. It didn't. I was no longer able to sleep because I suffocated every time I laid horizontally. I went to bed every night with my pillows propped up. I made an appointment to see my oncologist since I had no other options at that point.

In retrospect, had my pulmonologist called me back and ordered another steroid prescription, I may not have gotten to the real problem. Another example of God mysteriously working on my behalf.

My oncologist's office made an appointment for me to have a CT scan the very next day and scheduled a return visit to go over the results. My oncologist was perplexed with the results. He said there were masses in my lung, but he wasn't sure if it was pneumonia or cancer. He sent me for a PET scan and told me to come back in two days. However, if the PET scan showed no metabolic activity indicating cancer, the nurse practitioner would let me know it was pneumonia and call in a prescription for antibiotics, and I should cancel the appointment.

The phone never rang.

I went to bed more disappointed than ever, praying harder than ever. For the first time, my mantra *take me or heal me* focused on healing. I wasn't ready to leave, to lose my thirteen-year battle. I'd just met the person I wanted to be with, the person I'd been searching for over the last two decades. I wasn't ready!

Meeting Bertrand had thrown me off guard in one way I wasn't expecting: it was *easy*. We folded into each other's lives as if we'd always been there. We got along with each other's families, routinely cooking meals in his state-of-the-art kitchen, hosting friends, and planning dinner parties. When you're with the right person, it's remarkably simple to fit that person into your life.

I had the most vivid dream that night after waiting for the phone to ring, one I couldn't shake off the next day. I dreamt I was with my Aunt Ellen at the library. When I walked outside, a nurse appeared before me in a dazzling white dress. I was almost blinded by how white it was, and in my dream all I could think was, *What dry-cleaning service does she use? My whites are never that bright.*

She told me, "Your scans are clear. Your lung is fine, and you're going to live a long, healthy life."

"But what about my lung? Isn't it collapsed?"

She repeated, "Your scans are clear. Your lung is fine, and you're going to live a long, healthy life."

I had a great feeling of relief while in the dream. But when I woke up, the relief dissolved. I knew that wasn't my fate. There had been no call. I confessed my fears to Bertrand, something I would never have shared with my parents out of a fear of scaring them, and without hesitation, he said, "We'll face it together."

Two days later, the oncologist informed me that cancer had spread into my *left* lung. I had prepared myself for the news that I was no longer in remission, but not this. My left lung was my good lung, the only one I had left, and now it was compromised. Additionally, a mass was blocking my windpipe on my right side, causing the breathing trouble and wheezing sounds. And worse, cancer had spread into my hip bone, making it Stage 4 yet again. It was more aggressive than initially thought, and I needed to start treatment soon. I had at least one month, but would not survive beyond a year without medical intervention. It was Dr. Spira who said this, the man who always shied away from giving a death sentence. I took it to heart.

Aunt Ellen was with me at the appointment, intently reading a pamphlet on long-term care options. "Without freaking my aunt out,"

I whispered to Dr. Spira, "DC is legalizing physician-assisted suicide. Is this something I should look into?"

Very sternly he replied, "No, we are not there yet."

Part of me breathed a sigh of a relief. Not a big sigh, as I only had the one working lung and it was now compromised. But I trusted Dr. Spira to tell me the truth.

"Will you let me know when we are? I'm kind of exhausted. I need some sort of resolution," I pleaded.

"I will," he replied.

He then gave me two options: a trial he had mentioned in the past or immunotherapy.

I was nervous about immunotherapy because of the possibility of developing pneumonitis. He said there was a slim chance and it should not be the reason I didn't choose that. I reminded him I always got rare side effects, and I had lost my hair on Brentuximab when no one else did. He nodded in agreement.

I asked more about the trial, and he answered all my questions. Ninety people had been enrolled so far, and all had responded favorably, most taking six months to enter remission, although some had taken up to a year. I told him I needed to think over my options, and he left the room to get a referral.

I told my aunt about my dream. She was elated and yelled out a shriek of joy, which confused me, since I was just diagnosed with cancer for the millionth time.

She explained. "The woman in white was not the nurse practitioner; she was an angel. God is reassuring you that you will live a long, healthy life."

Strengthened by her words and by my own surety that God would not bring someone like Bertrand into my life only to take me so soon, I vowed to keep fighting. When I first met Bertrand, I thought the likelihood of us going the distance was slim based on my experience with other relationships.

But each time I'd given him an out, told him he didn't have to stick around for this difficult and ugly journey, he looked at me and said, "Are you crazy? I'm not going anywhere. You are stuck with me."

That's what I'd wanted my entire life, and I'd found it in this incredible man. I emailed my doctor the next day and told him I had decided to join the trial.

I also came to another realization that day. Every time I returned to work full-time, I got sick again. I was working ten-hour days plus dealing with a lengthy commute, and I'd also become a real estate agent on the side. I believe all of the stress taxed my body.

After my previous relapse, I was forced to cut my hours to part time and put a hold on taking on any new real estate clients. I promised myself I would put my health first, even if it meant delaying the chance of getting promoted. I knew I would never be a chief at the office or leave the federal government to become a partner at some fancy firm.

I could accept that.

I had put my career and professional development first time and again, starting back in 2003 when I was initially diagnosed and I'd refused to take a year off of law school to concentrate on getting healthy. Almost twenty years later, that hard lesson was hitting home: my health comes first.

Since Hodgkin's is a cancer of the lymphatic system, I am interminably immunocompromised. Think about that: being prone to every sickness or disease at any moment. A common cold can send me to the hospital with pneumonia. I have to avoid children at all costs. Try explaining that to all your friends. "Sorry, I can't come over because your germ-magnet kids could kill me." I am not the first on any party invitation list. I also had to step down from sitting on the board for Christian Legal Aid since all of their clinics were held in homeless shelters and I could not risk being in that environment.

In addition to having the immune system of a newt, I am on nine different medications, each with its own side effects. First thing in the morning, I take Synthroid (synthetic hormone) since my thyroid gland was nuked when I completed radiation in 2004. I have to take that on an empty stomach and cannot consume any food or beverage for thirty minutes, or antacids or vitamins within four hours. Then I take three cardiac medicines to keep my heart rate down and to strengthen my heart muscle. Those three medications drop my blood sugar levels and my blood pressure, so I have to take them after I eat. I have dangerously low blood pressure, so I take half the normal dosage of each of those medications. I also take a steroid pill and use a steroid inhaler in the morning for the pulmonary fibrosis, and use a nebulizer with Albuterol and saline solution in the evening.

Then, half an hour before dinner, I take Protonix for the heartburn I developed from all the radiation in my body. It literally burned holes in my digestive tract. In the evening, I take two more heart pills and magnesium. I forget to take my meds on a regular basis, so I have three alarms set throughout the day to remind me. Mix in all the doctors' appointments for check-ups and prescription refills—oncologist, cardiologist, pulmonologist—and working has become a real challenge. Healing myself is my new full-time job. This is why I have to be selfish.

✝

While waiting to be added to the trial, I struggled with the thought of going through another long crucible of treatments. I was getting tired and prayed for it all to be over. I prayed that God would take the cancer from me, that I would go into my next scan, and the doctors would be amazed, scratching their heads at how the cancer had simply disappeared. I knew God was able to do this. He had the power, but He was refusing to do so for some reason.

And that was the real struggle. I wondered why. After all this suffering, why hadn't he relieved me from it? What cosmic lesson had I not yet learned? I'm a good student and usually much quicker at learning lessons.

I arrived at church early that Sunday, and in my anguish, I prayed for a sign that God heard me, and prayed again that He would heal me miraculously. In the past, the prayer *take me or heal me* had sounded like a request. Now, I felt like I was giving God an ultimatum. I'd been a good Christian, a good person. I wanted the rewards of my faith. I wanted a cure. I wanted it now.

The message of the sermon couldn't have been more opposite, yet strikingly appropriate.

"Yes, sometimes you go through hard times," Pastor Charlie said. "Your baby dies, your husband leaves, you're crippled and left in a wheelchair. God sees it, knows it, ordains it, yet He is with you . . . and promises to carry you through it. But . . . " Pastor Charlie paused and stepped down from the raised platform, drawing near the congregation. "What if God doesn't heal you? What if all the stuff you fear . . . actually becomes your reality?"

I knew in that moment God was talking to me. He was answering my prayer. I listened like never before.

Charlie told the congregation that when he had lost his own child, he had prayed and prayed and prayed, but his child still died.

"How do you pick out a casket and burial plot for your child . . . and still go on believing in God? I struggled like you might not believe. I couldn't open the Bible for nine months. I went almost a year without praying. But then I remembered, God never promised to shield me from hardship. He promised to lead me through it. He never told me He would save me from pain, but He would turn it into blessing. He doesn't do what we want Him to. He does what He knows we need Him to."

I knew the truth in that moment. I was not going to be spontaneously healed. My scan wouldn't come back clear. And that was okay. God was with me, and He had control. That's all the confirmation I needed in that moment, that He was still in control. He saw everything and knew the end from the beginning, that this was supposed to be part of my story all along. And it was all for my eternal benefit. I would either be equipped with the tools to survive, or I would die. To be honest, being called to heaven sounded surprisingly good at that point.

I closed my eyes as the words of the pastor filled me and soothed me, provided a healing touch to a heart as scared as it was scarred by the cancer eating away at my insides. I'd made it this far with God standing by my side. I could make it a little farther.

I did, however, remind God that He had sent me an angel, and she had given me the message I was going to live a long and healthy life.

I am human, after all.

CHAPTER 31

And the Cat Becomes the (Lab) Mouse

The drug was so new that it didn't have an official name. ACD-301 was the name on the trial paperwork I filled out while waiting to join—and there's tons of paperwork involved in a drug trial. My ejection fraction was lower than the drug company wanted, so it took six weeks to get approval; red tape and what-not. Only Dr. Spira's heavy lobbying convinced the drug company I was right for their trials, and they finally acquiesced. The best part was that only four centers in the entire country were administering this drug, and my doctor happened to be one of them. This center was the only one on the East Coast with access, and he had patients enrolled in the trial coming from as far as North Carolina every two weeks.

Since the chemotherapy was to be administered through my veins, my doctor insisted I have a port catheter implanted. I refused. I'd had a port before. With my bony clavicle, it constantly protruded and made sleeping almost impossible.

On my first day of treatment, twenty-eight vials of blood were taken, four every hour for seven hours to monitor my levels. I also had four EKGs and two physical exams—the rigors of a trial for a drug that had never been tested on humans. It was known to create rashes in the mice and some of the first humans in the trial, so they put me on steroids. This made me insanely hungry and interrupted my sleep patterns. I have always prided myself on being a marathon sleeper, sometimes clocking in as much as ten hours in a single night. With the steroids, I slept a maximum of four. But I had no other side effects from the chemo—no nausea, no hair loss, no neutropenia. Not at first at least.

For once, everything was going well.

A few days after beginning the trial, my doctor informed me that two people had developed Guillain–Barré syndrome, a rare neurological disorder that could be fatal. I didn't have any of the symptoms he described. It made me nervous that I might get this condition since I had a history of developing every rare side effect of every drug I ever tried and even had reactions no one ever anticipated.

But what scared me more was that I would be unable to continue with the study if there were more occurrences of it. I hated thinking in those terms—of not worrying about the health and well-being of other patients, but of how it would impact me. The selfishness of this disease varied in its manifestations, but did not wane over the course of the last fifteen years. Still, I prayed. For all of us involved.

The FDA did partially close down the study and divided the participants into three groups. The patients who'd only had one treatment, like me, had to decide if they wanted to continue. If these patients continued, they would have to sign a new medical waiver. They temporarily closed off the study to new participants, and the participants who received more than one treatment could continue without disruption. I was thankful for my timing and jumped at the opportunity to sign my life away.

After a two-week delay, I completed the necessary paperwork and got my second treatment. After this, I was told I needed a PET scan and would have to show a partial response, some improvement, to continue with the study. If there was no response, it would not be worth the risk of continuing. The tumors needed to have shrunk by two-thirds. I apprehensively did the scan.

My response was remarkable, even better than they'd hoped. The tumors had shrunk 75 percent.

Good news lasts for only so long, and after my third treatment, I had double vision for a week. I emailed my doctor at 10 p.m. one night, and he immediately responded that I should get a brain MRI. I got it the very next day, and the scan was negative. Then I saw an ophthalmologist, who said I was in the clear. My cardiologist said my heart medications could cause double or blurry vision, and it was not the chemotherapy. Once all the doctors were on board, my oncologist cleared me for my next treatment.

Throughout treatments, nurses had trouble finding my veins until finally, having had enough, they informed me they would no longer administer any more drugs until I got a port. The nursing coordinator put in a referral to have the port inserted three weeks before my next treatment to give me enough time to heal from the soreness. Two and a half weeks later, I received a voicemail from the radiologist at 4:55 p.m. on Friday canceling my 7 a.m. Monday procedure. The doctor did not feel comfortable performing this procedure in the clinic on someone with my cardiac and pulmonary issues. He preferred the hospital setting. Suffice to say, by the next scheduled treatment on Wednesday, I still did not have a port.

I arrived for treatment and explained the situation to the nurses. Thankfully, they agreed to proceed and were able to administer the chemotherapy. It only took seven pokes, but afterward, my veins were so damaged that they could not draw blood. My veins were burning and had collapsed. I still have a noticeable scar from that afternoon. Eventually, I had the port inserted, and subsequent treatments went smoother.

A few days after that treatment, I developed a fever of 102°F and was instructed to go to the emergency room. My experience with trips to the emergency room did not instill a sense of confidence, and I was reluctant to put myself through an ordeal that would be taxing both mentally and physically. I had little energy to spare and even less patience.

However, upon examination, they discovered I was both septic and neutropenic, and diagnosed me with pneumonia; I promptly received my first round of antibiotics. Additional rounds of drugs were to be administered every twelve hours.

The ER doctor admitted me to the cancer wing, where I heard of a policy I had never before encountered. They refused to administer any fluids through the ports, maintaining that the risk of infection was much higher when this device was used. What a great irony!

If you think about it, cancer patients have ports because they have damaged, collapsed, sclerosed veins that make administering fluids and drawing blood a near impossibility. Just a few days ago, I had been forced to have a port inserted and now the hospital wouldn't use it. It seemed a perfect metaphor for the Catch-22 of my existence, and had I not been feeling so lousy, I might have found it amusing.

So, after three different nurses pricked me several times, I *requested* as politely but firmly as possible, that they use my port. Only the nurse in charge could access the port, however, and she was nowhere to be found. I asked to speak to the attending physician.

Hours later, the attending still had not come by my room. By 11 a.m., I still hadn't received my second dose of antibiotics. I was supposed to have received it three hours earlier. It wasn't until 1 p.m. that the attending finally came and received a complete and unfiltered earful. I wasn't trying to be unreasonable or unkind or uncooperative. I was trying to get better and the thing standing between me and that goal was the staff at the hospital charged with getting me better.

She explained that "due to the complications with administering the medication," my antibiotic regimen had to be changed. She warned me that the new regimen would make me nauseous because it was a continuous IV and I would need to remain in the hospital for an extra two days. Were they kidding? There was no way I was going to subject myself to two more days of their care.

I refused, and requested to be released under the care of my oncologist, Dr. Spira, for the next two doses of antibiotics. Reluctantly, and not for the first time, I was released against medical advice. I honestly thought, yet again, that I had a better chance of surviving on my own than in the care of the hospital.

It turns out that awful trip to the ER was not a total waste. While I was in the hospital that agonizing day, I started working on my smartphone application to help students study for the bar exam. Back when I was studying for the exam in 2010, I came up with the idea of creating a game similar to *Taboo*. Fast forward to 2018: after being home for two weeks and having grown tired of TV, I had evolved my game idea into an iPhone app.

After surviving these setbacks, I went in to see my oncologist and learned that I had, once again, entered into remission. The timing could not have been better since, during that same visit, I learned I would be unable to continue treatments due to the symptoms I had developed, symptoms the other people in the trial—not even the lab mice—had not developed. It was too risky to continue.

It was no surprise to me. I always developed the rarest of side-effects from treatment. But it was frustrating that I seemed to have some cosmic need to almost die with every new round of treatment. I found myself asking "why" a lot. Why does God keep letting me get sick and barely escape death, time after time? I'm never fully healed, and never fully alive. I found myself falling back to my prayer.

Take me or heal me.

Old habits die hard.

Then, my doctor added this "tiny little damper." The trial had not resulted in finding a cure, and many people on the new drug had relapsed, and . . . the only cure would be . . . a bone marrow transplant.

As disappointing as that was, I was happy to take a break for a while from the constant, life-altering decision-making and intravenous medication. I went home and told Bertrand the news, and we celebrated my latest remission. And after we had enjoyed the moment, I told him something that had been on my mind since the beginning of the trial.

"When the cancer comes back—and it most likely will—I'm done with treatments." Like any good lawyer, I laid out my reasoning. "I've lived a long life. I've loved, traveled, and witnessed my niece and nephews grow. I've accomplished every goal I set out to achieve. Not many people can say they passed the New York bar exam on their first try, and created an iPhone app on top of that. I love you . . . but I'm sick of being poked and prodded." I paused, building up my own resolve because this next part was difficult. I told him, "I want to stay together as long as I'm healthy, but if I get sick again, I'll pack up my stuff and move back home with my parents to live out the rest of my days with them."

He was understanding. He said it was my right and my body, and that if he had gone through everything I had, he probably would have decided the same.

So, we just sat there and stared at each other in this bittersweet moment.

"You love me," I told him.

"I do. Always." The perfect response.

I had a plan, a plan I was happy with. I prayed for at least five more years. I still had much to see and do—and I finally had someone I wanted to do it with.

Life #9

CHAPTER 32

Be Careful What You Wish For

It came as no surprise that I relapsed again. Nine months after I went off the trial, I went for a regular check-up and found out I was no longer in remission. I was again faced with deciding between treatments with varying pros and cons, and degrees of likelihood . . . healing me or killing me. And rather than giving my doctor the same prepared speech I had given my boyfriend nine months earlier, once again, I found myself asking more questions about the side effects of immunotherapy.

What happened to me "sticking to my guns" and saying "enough is enough"?

My heritage happened to it. My childhood happened to it. It's in my DNA. I really can't quit. Jordanians have always had a propensity for survival. Throughout the centuries, our people have been persecuted and expelled from their homes. Being survivors runs in our very DNA. When I was faced with a 104-degree fever back in 2005, I chose life. When the opportunity to join the Brentuximab study came up, I chose life. When gasping for air with an anaphylactic reaction, I clung to life. Each time, when push came to shove, I fought back. I'm a fighter. I choose life.

My oh-so-selfless declaration nine months before that at thirty-eight I'd lived enough life? I was full of it.

There was one more element of my equation to consider—Bertrand. Never before did I have someone outside of my family whom I cared enough about to want to live for. I'm ashamed to admit I was actually a little resentful. Even when I told him my plan nine months before, I knew I was lying, and in my mind, I blamed him for being yet another person for whom I felt I had to "stick around." Someone who tipped me over to the *heal me* side of the ultimatum. What a foolish person I am sometimes!

Even with the specter of my news hanging over us, Bertrand and I fell easily into our pattern of life. As I'd said, we just fit together. Family. Friends. When you're with the right person you know, and my heart and mind felt at ease around Bertrand. There was only one logical next step for us.

We planned a trip to Croatia in August 2019, and in the back of my mind, I knew it would be *the* trip. It's not something I would admit out loud, but I knew this trip would be special. Adding to the excitement of our departure, my app, BARRED, launched to the public on the day we took off.

One afternoon, Bertrand planned an outing to the island of Hvar, an island known for its sunshine and fields of lavender, rosemary, sage, and thyme. We took the ferry over and had lunch at a mountaintop restaurant with spectacular views of the crystal waters. Sitting there, I couldn't imagine a more beautiful location, and as Bertrand reached into his pocket, all I could think was . . . NO! I'd envisioned my engagement for years and the photos that would capture the moment. I finally had hair and it was a tangled, sweaty mess!

Luckily (or not), Bertrand pulled out the ferry schedule and we made our way back to the hotel. Later that night, after a long shower and time in front of the mirror getting my hair and makeup just right, we went down to dinner.

Just as the elevator doors opened, Bertrand announced, "I forgot my wallet." He kissed me. "Go grab our table and I'll be right back."

Just as the sun was setting, right on cue, the waiter came over and tapped me on the shoulder. I looked, and he was holding a bottle of champagne. So, of course, my head spun around to Bertrand, who was down on one knee, the most brilliant four-carat dazzler of a ring in his hand.

I'll keep his exact words to myself, because some things are meant to be kept between a couple. But he is the most romantic man on the planet, and when the shock and joy receded enough, I fell into his arms and screamed, *Yes!* It was everything I'd ever dreamed of. *He* was everything I'd ever dreamed of.

We toasted with the champagne, called our families, and celebrated our first night as an engaged couple. Safe in his arms that night, I thanked God for bringing Bertrand into my life, realizing it was yet another lesson from God in being careful what you wish for. I'd wanted a person, someone to share everything—the highs, the lows, the in-betweens. And I'd found him.

I had to live for Bertrand as much as myself. It would be cruel to suddenly bring him into my life, let him become a part of the wild, chaotic journey, then decide to quit. I couldn't do that to him. I realized it put additional pressure on myself to fight.

Cancer is selfish. I didn't want to be.

It's not always an easy choice to make.

We were engaged for less than a year as I planned the dream wedding. We were going to elope to Portugal, to a beautiful chapel I'd found in the Douro wine valley. I had the dress, the chapel, and the officiant all lined up and ready to receive us. The intimate candlelight dinner menu was planned, each course paired with a different glass of wine. We'd return to a reception in the Hamptons with family and friends. The perfect ending to a perfect engagement. Then . . .

COVID.

So instead, on 10/10/2020, we celebrated in Bertrand's sister's backyard with just twelve people, plus our officiant. The pandemic derailed all my plans, but at least I got the date I wanted. You have to take the little wins when you can. It was intimate and beautiful, and while it wasn't everything I planned, it was everything I needed. I didn't get the wedding of my dreams, but I certainly got the marriage of my dreams.

My parents, sadly, couldn't make the ceremony, so Loren planned to walk me down the aisle. However, she became so overwhelmed with emotion that she could not stop crying, so I had to walk myself down the aisle. I'd done so much on my own over the previous eighteen years, why not this too!

I think that's one of the lessons I had to learn on this journey: Not everything happens the way you expect it to, or even want it to. But it can still happen.

Maybe I'm just destined for life. My nickname in Arabic, Bisseh, gives me nine lives. My last name, Bsharat, means "good news." From my rosy-cheeked birth to my immigration as an infant while ill, to battle after battle with cancer, heart failure, lung failure . . . I am still here. If that is not good news, I don't know what is! Both prophecies have been realized.

During my regularly scheduled follow-up visit, the doctor reported increased activity in my right lung—the troublemaker. He said it wasn't conclusive and we could not safely biopsy it without it causing more harm. Plus, he rationalized that if it was cancer, it was barely there and waiting three months wouldn't kill me. We opted to wait.

For the first time in my life, I waited patiently. The kitten had grown into a tiger, but now I'd reverted to a domesticated house cat. I'd found love and a partner. I was no longer fighting alone. I had someone with me in the trenches, fighting by my side, fighting with me and for me. So, I didn't stress or become anxious. I took those three months as a chance to enjoy every second of my life. I had Thanksgiving, Christmas, my birthday, and a new year to celebrate. My brother's wife was pregnant, and I couldn't wait to learn whether I would soon meet a new nephew or niece. Three months later, I got the cancer diagnosis, and would finally start the immunotherapy regimen I had been dancing around for years.

Before, the risk of side effects had been too great. Immunotherapy had always been held out as a last resort. It was a theme for me during treatment—if there was a side effect that was going to present itself, I was going to find it. For that reason, I'd avoided immunotherapy. Now, my last resort was my only resort.

But deep down, I knew my life was in God's hands, no matter what I did or what the doctors said, whether I did more chemo, holistic treatments, or nothing at all. I was going to live for the time God allotted me to live, and die when it was my time to die.

The news didn't throw my world out of orbit. It didn't send me into a flurry of grief and pain. I knew now what I had only grasped at before: *God has never left my side.* He was always there, fighting the battles with me. If doctors overlooked something, and they always did, God found a way to put the answer in my path. Every time I had needs, He had solutions, before I even knew I needed them. Sometimes it took years to see them, but they were always there.

Finding love softened me. Rediscovering my faith strengthened me.

Throughout this journey, I've been trying to figure out why this was happening to me. *What am I supposed to learn?* I kept asking the heavens. I honestly thought that once I knew this answer, I would have this epiphany, add this newfound knowledge to my life, and I'd be healed. Just add faith and stir! Healing!

I may never know why I am sick, but I know I have become more caring and compassionate through my sickness, and that is definitely good. I would never have thought to become an advocate for people with disabilities until I was one. I never thought I would be the voice for others who couldn't find their own, but now I strive to be. I want to help those who don't have the training or confidence I do, in the face of doctors who move through the world by their reputations and not by their deeds. I've come to understand my relationship with God better through all of this, and hope I can help others do the same. Maybe that is my purpose. It is one I can live with.

Or maybe my purpose was to be sick, but to do it fearlessly. To do all of this knowing God has my back and to share that knowledge with others: *He is always with us. He is walking with us, fighting for us. We are never alone.* So, we can fight our battles gracefully.

There is a listserv at my work where people can email Bible verses and daily devotions. One day, a man wrote that God's love for us is like a father's love for his child, only how much more does God love his children than an earthly father loves his? A father wants to give his children everything they need. He hates seeing them in pain and wants to erase it. Even more, God wants to take our pain away.

The man quoted the Scripture, "By His stripes we are healed," referring to how God took away all disease in the world through the act of Jesus dying on the cross. The man continued to say that "disease, then, is not a part of God's perfect plan for us, so if we pray very hard, then all diseases will be healed."

When I first developed in my faith, I used to believe that. If God loves me, He will cure me. If God loves me, He will take away this cancer.

But I don't anymore. And it's not because I don't believe He can. I do believe He is able, but I also believe our life on Earth is only temporary, and it's the life that comes *after* that fulfills the promise of being truly healed.

For the past two decades, I followed His rules: I studied, I believed, I practiced what I preached, I did every single thing He asked of me. I thought surely that would guarantee me a cure. I thought a cure was a fair exchange for my obedience. But I slowly realized the Bible never promises a cure; it never promises us freedom from pain or to live an easy life. In fact, it tells us the opposite. It warns us we will have a life full of pain, but that God will be there with us through it all. I now understand

I will have heartbreak and trauma in this life—but I also know I do not have to go through it alone. He will be with me, and He will not forsake me in my storms. I learned the hard way that disease is not from God, but He allows it and promises to lead us through to the end, whenever that may be. My life, your life—for all its pains and imperfections, we are part of His perfect plan.

As I matured in my faith, I realized living in a tragedy does not mean I am living without God's blessing. God can love and bless me, but still allow bad things to happen. The blessing comes from Him being with me.

Moses endured the hardships of wandering through the desert for forty years, only to be denied entry to the Promised Land. Not fair! Neither was it fair when Isaac went blind and his son betrayed him, nor when Sarah had to wait ninety-nine years to bear a child, at which point God requested for that child to be sacrificed. Was it fair when Joseph was sold into slavery by his own brothers and wrongly accused and sent to prison? Don't get me started on Job, or Jesus.

No one in the Bible lived a life free of suffering or injustice. And if they lived like that, being God's chosen people, why should my life be different? I believe we have suffering so we can stay near to God. Faith wouldn't be faith if only good things happened.

Sometimes, God does not heal us. And when we read "by His stripes we are healed." I believe it's a spiritual healing, not a physical one.

I see that difference in me now.

Physically, I am more broken than I was eighteen years ago, but emotionally and spiritually, I am a new person, made whole and strong. While on this journey, my faith has been tested many times through the people who were supposed to take care of me. But while I've been here, there have been many ways God has lifted me up through the kindness of others—from driving me to appointments and sending me care packages, to introducing me to a convenience store owner who would later open up his home.

I look back on the agonizing conversations I had with so many different doctors, searching for the answer. *The elusive cure.* But I now see that, whether I chose more chemotherapy, holistic treatments in Mexico or Timbuktu, or nuking my body until I glowed in the dark, I was going to survive as long as God decided He wants me around. All the sleepless nights trying to decide, and the conversations where I kicked myself for choosing the wrong option, were moot. I am where I am meant to be, until God calls me home.

He has shown me miracles: giving me the intuition I needed to stop treatments and eat certain foods, helping me to meet people at parties, to miss trains and stumble into bookstores, assigning a massage therapist to live next door to me, enrolling me in a study that is offered in only four states nationwide and is only twenty minutes from my house . . . the list goes on and on.

I was never alone.

My faith was always there, just like God. I just didn't understand it, and keeping my disease a secret for so many years kept me from realizing my purpose and identity, and recognizing God's presence in my life. Talking about my experiences led me to learning the lessons I needed, and sharing them cultivated my growth.

I know my physical healing will be fully granted in Heaven, when God decides it's time for me to shuffle off this mortal coil and I will no longer be burdened with the shackles of an earthly body. The safety and strength of that knowledge is why I can relax from Bisseh the Tiger to Bisseh the House Cat. *His* stripes have healed me; not my tiger stripes. I no longer need claws to fight to survive. I choose to allow my faith in God to carry me through, with Bertrand by my side, whatever may come.

Don't get me wrong; I still have my moments. I still struggle to find it all joyous. But I have much to be grateful for. I have supportive family and friends, a wonderful loving husband, and a great job with fantastic benefits. But if I lost my hair again, would I say, "No problem. I'll just get another sexy wig?" We'll see. Some days are harder than others. On the hard days, I cry a lot and eat junk food. But on most days, I see that God is in control. And more so, I rely on my community to rally behind me.

For a long time, I worried I was in a codependent relationship with cancer. I worried I didn't know how to be cancer free. There was always this apprehensiveness when I was in remission. I was like a long-tailed cat in a room full of rocking chairs. I felt safe with cancer. Who would I be without it? Having *it* took the worrying and wondering away.

Now, I don't fear the cancer or the remission because I see God in every step. I no longer worry about whether I will be cured. I may never find the cure to my sickness, but I have found something infinitely better.

I have found peace in the shadow of the mountain. I learned that, rather than having me circle the same mountain, God was in fact moving it.

They say insanity is doing the same thing over and over again but expecting a different outcome. So why is it that every time I am in remission and stop the drugs, I am surprised that the cancer comes back? I think that's when faith comes in—faith that it will be different this time. Faith is confidence in what we hope for and the assurance that God is working, even though we cannot see it. Faith knows that no matter what the situation—in our lives or in someone else's—God is in control. I may never be free from this cancer, but I have hope I will, and the knowledge that the good Lord is able. Therefore, I have faith that I will see another day.

I once read that hope is not insurance that we won't have troubles in our lives. It's an assurance that God will be with us, however long or difficult the journey.

I may always have cancer, but it doesn't have me anymore.

Take me or heal me, I no longer pray.

I am healed.

Postscript

You didn't think my story would end there, did you? I'm like a Timex or the Energizer Bunny.

Bertrand and I settled into life after our wedding. After having to postpone my dream wedding, I watched the news closely when the new COVID vaccine made the news. My health history put me close to the top of the list of early recipients, and I received my first vaccine in February and my second dose in March 2021.

I had some mild symptoms associated with the vaccine, but I didn't think anything of it because they went away in due course. In early May, I went in for a scheduled PET scan, followed by my monthly blood work and treatment. This was something I had been doing for two years; I could do it with my eyes closed. It seemed that on this day, everyone was doing their jobs with their eyes closed. It was a comedy of errors.

The PET scan ran late, so of course, then I was late for my follow-up at the lab. I arrived at the lab for the routine bloodwork and was told that the PET scan results had been received. After the blood draws, I went in to see the doctor, but there were no PET scan results. We really couldn't have a meaningful conversation, but things had been status quo, and we decided to stay the course. I was sent for my treatment; while I sat in the chair I texted and emailed the radiology office trying to get my PET scan results. If, by some chance, the PET showed an abnormality, my doctor would want to know for certain before giving me a drug that costs $28,000 and no longer working.

At the very last moment (the nurse was hovering just inches away with the needle), my PET scan results arrived.

It's strange the power of a few seconds. Life before and after. I'd lived it so often you'd think I'd be numb to the power of the words, but getting hit by that Mac truck never gets any easier.

The cancer was back.

I stopped the nurse. I tried to remember how to breathe. This wasn't supposed to happen. Not again. I'd paid the piper over and over. I tried to will the clock to wind back, to unread those words, to return to the blissful ignorance of a few moments ago. But I couldn't. Bertrand's face filled my head. My parents. My siblings. Nieces and nephews. Friends. So many faces.

I'd said it before that I wouldn't fight, but we know how that turned out. I knew that wasn't an option anymore. I had people to live for.

I jumped up from the treatment chair, a woman on a mission, filled with the determination of eighteen years of fighting and winning against this damned disease. I stalked the halls of the clinic, looking for Dr. Spira. I must have resembled a mad woman because everyone got out of my way as I plowed through the halls. Apparently, I made quite the impression. So much for that inner peace I'd been working on all those years.

When I finally found him, I shoved my phone in his face.

"It's back." I handed him the phone and let him read the words himself. I think he was as shocked as I. "Now what?"

He was quiet, the news stealing the words from his lips as much as they had lit a fire in my belly. "Let's go back to my office. I need to think."

Thinking was good, but I wanted a game plan.

Back in his office, he told me about a mild version of chemo called Gemcitabine that was a possibility, but he still wanted time to think and review the PET scan. That it had gone straight to Stage 4 in my spleen was out of character. In the world of cancer, out of character was not good news.

On that bright note, I asked the question doctors hated. "How long?"

I felt like life had just started for me. Married. Happy. I hadn't yet gone on my honeymoon. I still had things to do, and cancer was not on the agenda.

Dr. Spira looked at me over the thick tome that constituted my medical file. "I'm not going to answer that." He put down the file. "I want time to think, look over the latest research. Review what treatments you have already done." There were no new drugs in the pipeline, that much I knew. Things changed slowly in the area of cancer research, but I tried not to think of the word hopeless. "Go home," he told me. "We'll talk soon."

Somehow, I managed to get home—it's honestly a blur. I walked into the apartment and was met first by an excited ball of fluff, our new puppy Kaia. Over Kaia's excited yaps, I could hear Bertrand in his office, and he called out, "How was treatment?"

I didn't answer, completely overwhelmed at facing the start of another leg on this journey. I thought of all the people who had stood by me in the past and all the people I had now. I thought of Bertrand and the life we'd just started to build. I wanted to scream and shout at the unfairness of it all. But I didn't.

My quiet entrance alone, I'm sure, alerted Bertrand that something was wrong. I'm loud when I walk into a room—the Macy's Thanksgiving Day parade is sedate compared to me. Today, I was quiet.

Bertrand came around the corner, and I could tell he knew without me saying a word. I don't know what my face looked like but his was a mask of complete devastation.

We sat down, snuggled so close together I couldn't tell where I ended and he began. He tried to be strong, so I didn't have to be, and he said every right thing anyone wants to hear from the one they love in such a situation. I married such a total rock star. I'd never loved him more.

"I know you're tired." He traced circles and hearts on the back of my hand. Endless love. "Tired of treatments and the uncertainty and losing your hair and tired of fighting. But we haven't had our honeymoon yet. I need you to live for me, for us. My future depends on you being alive."

While this is what I was fearful of when I got married, of being asked to put someone else's well-being before my own when my health was so precarious, it was also the reason I got married. I wanted someone to walk with me and walk beside me, to share the highs and lows.

So, sitting there wrapped in love, it was an easy decision. We did the most natural thing given our situation—we took the dog for a walk.

Bertrand and I made plans to go in and talk to the doctor on the following Monday. At the office, we discussed the options.

Dr. Spira went into more detail about the drug he referred to the week before, Gemcitabine. He explained it is a long-term maintenance chemo program that involved treatment three weeks on, one week off. It was more aggressive than my existing treatment that had me one week on, three weeks off. It was a mild form of chemo but would necessitate my looking at either medical retirement or FMLA. The career I'd worked so hard for was once again falling prey to the predatory cancer.

"And if I do nothing?" Here I was again, asking the question doctors hated to answer. I saw Bertrand stiffen when I said the words, and truthfully, they hurt worse to say this time around. I had something to live for. I reached over and took Bertrand's hand. I didn't want to give up.

Dr. Spira closed my file and put it aside. "My best guess is two to five years." He crossed his arms and took a deep breath. "But that isn't an option for you. You got married. I want to give you twenty-five more years. That's my game plan. I just need you to work with me."

He looked so determined sitting there in his starched white coat. It must have been contagious because Bertrand wore a similar expression. I closed my eyes and said a prayer of thanks to God for putting two such stubborn men in my life.

I asked Dr. Spira if I could take three months to wrap my head around the news and decide next steps. We had some family obligations coming soon, and I didn't want to be in the middle of chemo and radiation while traveling. There was also a tiny part of me that was still my parents' daughter: keep the news private. There would be no doubt what was going on if we attended these events while I was in the middle of chemo.

"I'm not in favor of the hiatus, but waiting won't kill you," he said with a smile.

Cancer jokes. I guess sometimes laughter really is the best medicine.

At home, Bertrand voiced his support for starting chemo now. His niece was getting married in California in three months, so I'd be starting chemo just as we were leaving for the wedding, if I waited.

"If you start now, you'll be in remission by then." I loved his positive outlook.

He also dived into online research, looking for alternative reasons for an enlarged spleen. I knew this was part of his processing. He was in denial. Having traveled down this road many times, I recognized the signs. He didn't want to accept the diagnosis or the potential outcome.

He did find an interesting article that connected the COVID vaccine to false-positive PET scans for enlarged lymph nodes under the arm and anecdotal evidence for increased size in the spleen, which is exactly what my PET scan had shown. Ever the armchair doctor, we sent it on to Dr. Spira, but he said it wasn't related. Regardless, we decided to wait a month and redo my PET scan. If my cancer was aggressive and followed the normal path, it would grow. If my PET scan results were a reaction to the vaccine, the positive reaction would decrease.

As I finish writing this postscript, I'm waiting on the repeat PET scan. It's also why this is called a postscript and not an epilogue. This is not the end of my journey; I plan to keep adding to the story.

But I do know this: whatever happens, I have my faith in God, I have Bertrand, and I have my family. My story is far from over.

✝

Taita, Jedo, Uncle Eric, and Rana: "What we once loved, we can never lose. For all that we love deeply becomes part of us."

– *Helen Keller*

Glossary of Terms

ABVD: Adriamycin + Bleomycin + Vinblastine + Dacarbazine is a chemotherapy regimen used in the first-line treatment of Hodgkin's Lymphoma.

Against Medical Advice: a medical term commonly used in all health institutions when a patient decides to leave the hospital against the advice of the doctor. In order to refuse care, the patient must meet the following criteria: 1. The patient is over the age of eighteen years. 2. The patient exhibits no evidence of an altered level of consciousness or impaired judgment from alcohol or drug ingestion. 3. The patient understands the nature of the medical condition, as well as the risks and consequences of refusing care.

AMA: see Against Medical Advice

Anemia: is defined as a low number of red blood cells, which is detected through a routine blood test showing low hemoglobin or hematocrit levels. Hemoglobin is the main protein in red blood cells; it carries oxygen and delivers it throughout the body. With anemia, hemoglobin levels will be low too, and if they are low enough, the tissues or organs may not receive enough oxygen. Symptoms of anemia include fatigue or shortness of breath.

Blood Ozone Therapy: ozone therapy involves using ozone gas ($O3$ or trioxygen), a potent form of oxygen, as a disinfectant agent that is introduced into affected areas of the body via IV. Ozone therapy, also known as autohemotherapy, takes some blood, enriches it with ozone, and cycles that ozonated blood directly back into the bloodstream. The

ozonated blood then delivers oxygen-rich nutrients to every part of
the body, thereby boosting the immune system response and helping
reduce the stress on the lungs.

Cancer: a disease in which some of the body's cells grow uncontrollably
and spread to other parts of the body. Cancer can start almost anywhere in
the human body, which is made up of trillions of cells. Normally, human
cells grow and multiply through a process called cell division to form new
cells as the body needs them. When cells grow old or become damaged, they
die, and new cells take their place. However, sometimes this orderly process
breaks down, and abnormal or damaged cells grow and multiply when
they shouldn't. These cells may form tumors, which are lumps of tissue.
Tumors can be cancerous or non-cancerous (benign). Cancerous tumors
spread into—or invade—nearby tissues and travel to distant places in the
body to form new tumors (a process called metastasis).

Candida cleansing: a diet that eliminates sugar, white flour, yeast,
and cheese, based on the theory that these foods promote candida
overgrowth. Candida is a yeast, which is a type of fungus. Candida
is typically found in the gastrointestinal tract, but an overgrowth can
exacerbate existing gastrointestinal diseases and other infections once it
spreads to vital organs or the bloodstream.

Cardiomyopathy: a progressive disease of the myocardium, or heart
muscle. In most cases, the heart muscle is enlarged, thick or rigid,
and unable to pump blood to the rest of the body as well as it should.
In rare instances, diseased heart muscle tissue is replaced with scar
tissue. Cardiomyopathy can lead to heart failure. Treatment includes
medications, surgically implanted devices, heart surgery, or, in severe
cases, a heart transplant.

CT Scan: Computed Tomography Scan (formerly known as Computed
Axial Tomography or CAT scan) is a medical imaging technique
used to get detailed images of the body noninvasively for diagnostic
purposes. This diagnostic tool combines a series of X-ray images taken
from different angles around the body and uses computer processing

to create cross-sectional images (slices) of the bones, blood vessels, and soft tissues inside the body. CT scan images provide more detailed information than plain X-rays do.

Defibrillator: devices that restore a normal heartbeat by sending a dose of electric current (often called a counter-shock) to the heart, which depolarizes a large amount of the heart muscle, ending the dysrhythmia. Defibrillators can also restore the heart's beating if the heart suddenly stops. A small battery-powered device placed in the chest to monitor the heart rhythm and detect irregular heartbeats. The device then sends electric shocks via one or more wires connected to the heart to fix an abnormal heart rhythm if detected.

Echocardiogram: also known as an echo, an echocardiogram uses sound waves to produce images of the heart, creating a graphic outline of the heart's movement. This common test allows the doctor to see the heart beating and pumping blood in order to identify heart disease. During an echo test, an ultrasound (high-frequency sound waves) from a hand-held wand is placed on the chest, which provides pictures of the heart's valves and chambers and helps the sonographer evaluate the strength of the pumping action of the heart.

Ejection Fraction: (EF) is a measurement doctors use to calculate the percentage of blood flowing out of the ventricles with each contraction of the heart. EF refers to how well the left or right ventricle pumps blood with each heartbeat and is expressed as a percentage. An EF that is below normal can be a sign of heart failure. Measuring EF can help doctors figure out whether certain heart problems exist, especially one type of heart failure.

Epstein-Barr Virus: (EBV) one of the most common human viruses in the world. It spreads primarily through saliva. EBV can cause infectious mononucleosis, also called mono, and other illnesses. Most people will get infected with EBV in their lifetime and will not have any symptoms.

Graft Versus Host Disease: (GVHD) a potentially serious complication of allogeneic stem cell transplantation. During allogeneic stem cell transplantation, a patient receives stem cells from a donor or donated umbilical cord blood. GVHD occurs when the donor's T cells (the graft) view the patient's healthy cells (the host) as foreign and attack and damage them. Symptoms can range from mild to severe and often include skin inflammation, jaundice, and GI discomfort, to life-threatening with multiple organ failure.

Hemoglobin: the iron-containing protein molecule in red blood cells that carries oxygen from the lungs to the body's tissues and returns carbon dioxide from the tissues back to the lungs. Hemoglobin is made up of four protein molecules (globulin chains) that are connected together. When someone has insufficient red blood cells or the ones they have do not work properly, the body is left short of the oxygen it needs to function. This condition is called anemia.

Hodgkin's Lymphoma: also known as Hodgkin's Disease or Hodgkin Lymphoma (HL), this is a type of lymphoma, which is a blood cancer that starts in the lymphatic system. The lymphatic system helps the immune system get rid of waste and fight infections. HL originates in white blood cells that help protect the body from germs and infections. These white blood cells are called lymphocytes. In people with HL, these cells grow abnormally and spread beyond the lymphatic system. As the disease progresses, it makes it more difficult for the body to fight infections. Between 8,000 and 9,000 people are diagnosed with Hodgkin's Lymphoma in the United States each year. The disease is most frequently diagnosed among people ages 20-34.

Laetrile: also known as Amygdalin, is a compound that has been used as a treatment for people with cancer. Laetrile is a bitter substance found in fruit pits, such as apricots, raw nuts, lima beans, clover, and sorghum. It makes hydrogen cyanide, which is changed into cyanide when taken into the body and can be used to kill certain cancer cells.

Lymphoma: a cancer of the lymphatic system, which is part of the body's germ-fighting network. The lymphatic system includes the lymph nodes (lymph glands), spleen, thymus gland, and bone marrow. Lymphoma can affect all those areas as well as other organs throughout the body. Many types of lymphoma exist. The main subtypes are Hodgkin's Lymphoma (formerly called Hodgkin's Disease) and Non-Hodgkin's Lymphoma.

MVP: Mitomycin-C, Vinblastine, and Platinum (Cis-Platin) chemotherapy cocktail is an intravenous treatment for certain cancers, including lung cancer, mesothelioma, and breast cancer. It is considered a salvage chemotherapy, which is given to patients who do not respond to other chemotherapy regimens.

Neulasta: a prescription medicine used to help reduce the chance of infection due to a low white blood cell count in people with certain types of cancer or those who receive anti-cancer medicines such as chemotherapy. It is a colony-stimulating factor, which is a man-made form of a protein that stimulates the growth of white blood cells, used to decrease the incidence of infection by treating neutropenia, a lack of certain white blood cells.

Neutropenia: a condition where there is a lower-than-normal level of neutrophils, a type of white blood cell, in the blood. While all white blood cells help the body fight infections, neutrophils are important for fighting certain infections, especially those caused by bacteria. Neutropenia might happen due to an infection but can also result from cancer treatment.

PET Scan: Positron Emission Tomography, also called PET imaging, is a diagnostic examination that measures metabolic activity of the cells by taking images of the body based on the detection of radiation from the emission of positrons. Positrons are tiny particles emitted from a radioactive substance administered to the patient via radiotracers that are injected into the veins.

PFT: see Pulmonary Function Test

Port a catheter: also known as Port-A-Cath, is a device that contains a port—a small, round reservoir covered with a plastic membrane—and a catheter. The port is implanted just below your skin, while the catheter runs under the skin into a large vein. A needle can easily puncture the plastic membrane to deliver medication such as chemotherapy or withdraw blood.

Procrit: a prescription medicine used to treat anemia. People with anemia have a lower–than–normal number of red blood cells (RBCs). Procrit works like the human protein called erythropoietin to help your body make more RBCs. Procrit is used to reduce or avoid the need for RBC transfusions.

Pulmonary Fibrosis: a lung disease that occurs when lung tissue becomes damaged and scarred. This thickened, stiff tissue makes it more difficult for the lungs to work properly. As pulmonary fibrosis worsens, the scar tissue can destroy the normal lung and make it hard for oxygen to get into the blood, causing shortness of breath. There is no cure for this disease.

Pulmonary Function Test: (PFTs) are noninvasive tests that show how well the lungs are working. The tests measure lung volume, capacity, rates of flow, and gas exchange. This information can help health care providers diagnose and decide the treatment of certain lung disorders. The most basic test is spirometry, which measures the amount of air the lungs can hold, and also measures how forcefully one can empty air from the lungs.

Sepsis: a potentially life-threatening condition that occurs when the body's response to an infection damages its own tissues. When the infection-fighting processes turn on the body, they cause organs to function poorly and abnormally. Sepsis may progress to septic shock, which is a dramatic drop in blood pressure that can lead to severe organ problems and death. Early treatment with antibiotics and intravenous fluids improves chances for survival.

Resources

Leukemia & Lymphoma Society: www.LLS.org
The Leukemia & Lymphoma Society is the world's largest voluntary
health agency dedicated to blood cancer. LLS's mission is to cure
leukemia, lymphoma, Hodgkin's disease, and myeloma, and to improve
the quality of life of patients and their families.

Samfund: www.thesamfund.org
The Samfund provides support to young adults who are struggling
financially because of cancer. Through direct financial assistance and
free online support and education, they help young adults survive and
move forward with their lives after cancer.

Make-A-Wish: www.wish.org
The Make-A-Wish Foundation is a 501(c)(3) nonprofit organization
founded in the United States that helps fulfill the wishes of children
with critical illnesses between the ages of two-and-a-half and eighteen.

Gilda's Club: www. Gildasclub.org
Gilda's Club is a community organization for people with cancer, their
families, and friends. Local chapters provide meeting places where
those who have cancer, their families, and friends can join with others
to build emotional and social support as a supplement to medical care.
Free of charge and a nonprofit, Gilda's Club chapters offer support
and networking groups, lectures, workshops, and social events in a
nonresidential, home-like setting. The club was named in honor of the
original *Saturday Night Live* cast member Gilda Radner, who died of
ovarian cancer in 1989.

About the Author

Rinad Bsharat was born in Mafraq, Jordan. Her family immigrated to New York in 1980 and eventually settled in Harrison, New York, where Rinad was raised with her two brothers and sister.

She earned a BS at The George Washington University and a law degree at The City University of New York School of Law. Rinad works as a lawyer with the federal government and is a licensed realtor in the state of Virginia. She is also the Founder and Chief Executive Officer of BARRED, a gaming app aimed at helping law students to study for the bar exam.

A nine-time cancer survivor and an avid traveler, Rinad is a proud aunt to eight nieces and nephews. She currently lives in northern Virginia with her husband, Bertrand, and mini-Husky, Kaia.

CPSIA information can be obtained
at www.ICGtesting.com
Printed in the USA
BVHW030530011221
622872BV00012B/598/J